Canary in a Bubble

Summer Lei'Dawn
2021

Library of Congress Catalog Number (LCCN): 2021918623

ISBN: 978-1-7378403-1-2 (Softcover)
ISBN: 978-1-7378403-0-5 (Hardcover)
ISBN: 978-1-7378403-2-9 (Digital)

Contact information:
E-mail: CanaryinaBubble@gmail.com
Website: www.CanaryinaBubble.com

Merita Gail Publishing
P.O Box 335
Moundville, AL. 35474

Dedication / Acknowledgement.

To the ones who feel forgotten.

To the ones who feel afraid.

To the ones wandering the valleys in hopes of finding Grace.

To the ones who stayed and to the ones who left.

To the one who carried me up the mountain when I couldn't catch a breath.

To the Good Samaritans who saw worth in trying to save a life and to the Priest and Levites who just walked on by.

- Summer Lei Dawn

Contents

Intro

As I woke up from being under anesthesia from surgery for endometriosis, I could feel my heart racing and my skin burning as if I were blistering in the scalding sun. I could not open my eyes or find the strength to call out for help, and if that weren't scary enough, I could feel my throat slowly starting to swell. As the panic set in, I was finally able to muster up the strength to let out a loud groan, but it was suppressed by the sound of a very hectic recovery room. *This is the end,* I thought to myself, until I heard the sweet small voice of a nurse calling out for medication because a patient in recovery was having an allergic reaction. That's when I felt the warmth of her hand grasp my arm as she assured me that everything was going to be okay. She then administered IV Benadryl, and within moments the burning on my skin and the swelling calmed down. I had never encountered an allergic reaction so severe that it could leave someone so helpless, but little did I know it was only the beginning of an extremely dramatic battle that was yet to come.

During this time in my life, I was around the age of twenty-three; I loved spending all of my free time outdoors, whether it was sitting outside early in the morning, sipping on a nice hot creamy mocha while reading my devotional, or sitting down by the warm campfire on a beautiful fall night with my family and friends while listening to the crickets play their song under the big starry sky.

Those were the days—the days when I remember feeling normal and not like an outsider looking in—but soon those mornings filled with the aroma of luscious chocolate mocha and those starry nights spent laughing by the fire all started slowly fading away to what seemed like a distant memory.

A few months had passed after experiencing my very first anaphylactic reaction that occurred during surgery, and I was so grateful to be alive. I walked away from that experience thinking it would be a once-in-a-lifetime event which truly opened my eyes to see the truth of just how fast things can spin out of control and just how precious life really is.

Chapter 1

In the Beginning

I slowly started to notice very weird symptoms that ranged from joint pains all the way to anaphylactic symptoms. Looking back at just how much time has gone by since the beginning of this battle amazes me, because it seems like yesterday, but at the same time it feels as if it was a lifetime ago.

I remember one day I was in the shower, trying to pick up the shampoo bottle to squirt a small amount into my hand, and as I squeezed it, an intense pain shot through my wrist. It felt as if the joints in my wrist were being cut open from the inside out.

As time passed, I started noticing that my skin would randomly burn, itch, and turn a bright shade of red, and my throat would randomly swell. Being as active as I was, it was difficult to pinpoint during that time what exactly was causing my symptoms, so my doctor suggested that I see an allergist.

I made an appointment, and the allergist drew labs and ordered blood work to check for any sign of unknown allergies. The results showed that I was allergic to red and yellow dyes, but everything else was normal. I was surprised to learn I had an allergy to something so widespread, since synthetic dyes are used in basically everything from our food supplies to our hygiene products and more. I was sure that I consumed a sizeable amount of artificial dyes daily.

Because synthetic dyes are in so many products, I had to research information on my own online to learn more (the doctor only had so many answers), and I'm sure at that moment in time I probably looked like a deer caught in the headlights.

The more I looked into it, the more I learned some truly disturbing facts, such as:

1. Most synthetic dyes are made from petroleum, which is a crude oil product that is used to make things like diesel fuel, plastic, asphalt and gas. Now imagine that same product in your dyed breakfast cereal.

2. Artificial dyes come with an entire list of health concerns of their own, such as being linked to causing hyperactivity, hypersensitivity, and mood disorders in children.

This one hit home with me, as I have had ADHD since I was a child, and because of that I was forced to take Adderall and Ritalin, which I absolutely hated because it caused me not to feel like my happy self. I truly believe a diet change to eliminate all artificial dyes would have helped me better than either of the medications that were being pushed at me.

I have seen this in my son as well. Give him a chocolate chip cookie with artificial food dye in it and he will go bonkers, running around the room 90 to nothing, but if you give him an organic chocolate chip cookie, he is completely fine. The behavioral difference is astonishing to me.

3. Artificial dyes have been shown to cause cancerous tumors in mice and rats.

4. In 1990, Red #3 was discovered to actually be an animal carcinogen! Red #40, Yellow #5 and Yellow #6 have been shown to be contaminated with known carcinogens, which means that they can cause cancer, but for some reason the FDA thinks that certain levels are safe in our foods. But are they really?

Artificial dyes have also been linked to:

- Chromosomal damage
- Asthma and bronchitis
- Eczema
- Allergies
- A negative impact on vital organs.

- A disruption of the immune system because the molecules they contain attach to the proteins in our bodies.

Interestingly, several countries have bans on certain artificial dyes because of the health risks associated with them. Great Britain, for example, told the major food companies that they could no longer add the artificial dyes to their food products in the UK! After learning that they linked these synthetic dyes all over the world to health issues, I couldn't help but ask myself why anyone would pump this crap into our children's food, much less our own?

After all my research, I thought to myself, *Okay, maybe this is it. All I need to do is make a few changes to my diet and eat a little healthier.* But boy was I wrong.

Not too long after that I noticed new and more intense symptoms. For instance, if someone walked by with a strong perfume, it would rock my head so hard that I would become faint and dizzy with an unbelievable amount of brain fog, my skin would break out in hives and my tongue and throat would begin to swell. This started becoming a frequent issue anytime I came in contact with pesticides, herbicides, perfumes, food additives, candles, essential oils, air fresheners, laundry soap, cigarette smoke, and the list goes on and on.

The pesticides and herbicides became an enormous obstacle in my way, because not only was I reacting to it through environmental exposure, such as driving past a state truck spraying hazardous herbicides on the side of the road, but now it was causing my body to reject certain foods.

Here I was, once again learning about toxins in our food supplies the hard way, through sweat, tears and even blood. After several long hours of research, I learned some interesting facts, like:

- Up to 70% of nonorganic produce sold in the U.S. contains traces of pesticides even when washed.
- Pesticide levels have been detected in more than 90% of Americans' blood and urine.
- Pesticides like glyphosate, organophosphates and neonicotinoids have been detected in 100% of nonorganic applesauce and breakfast cereals.
- A study published by PIOS Medicine showed organophosphates at low levels cause brain damage in children and, interestingly enough, it was originally created as a nerve agent.

Pesticide exposure has also been linked to:

- Cancer
- DNA damage
- Endocrine disruption

- Reproductive issues
- Asthma and bronchitis
- Parkinson's disease
- Children exposed to pesticides have a greater risk of being diagnosed with ADHD and having a lower IQ, and studies have also shown children with indoor exposure have an increased risk of leukemia by 47% and lymphoma by 43%.

So, I couldn't help but ask myself again, "Why is this in our food supplies?"

That doesn't even begin to cover the additives in our food supplies that have been linked to hormone disruption, increased cancer risk and damage to the central nervous system!

One thing that overwhelmingly stood out to me was the fact that most of the breakfast cereals, pastries, cakes, candies, snacks and treats that were being marketed specifically toward children were full of these harmful ingredients!

No matter which way I look at it, there is no logical explanation why anyone with good intentions would ever add these harmful chemicals to our food supplies, especially when there are healthier options available.

Chapter 2

The Pass Around. Alpha Who?

I made another appointment with the allergist because the symptoms I was experiencing were becoming more frequent and unbearable, so she prescribed a few medications for me to try. She tried to explain that the medical community really doesn't know that much about the immune system and that sometimes things like this just happen and that she couldn't provide an answer as to what was causing it.

So, I came home and took the medications she had prescribed as directed, but I soon noticed side effects, such as a complete change in my moods, itchy sensations randomly happening across my body, and facial swelling. It seemed the longer I was on the medications, the worse the side effects became, so I eventually stopped taking the medications and decided that I needed to get a second opinion. By this time, my body had started reacting to all the non-organic food items I had tried so my husband started buying more organic foods to try, and at the onset it seemed to work—until it did not. Turns out foods with an organic label only need to be 95% organic, not 100% organic!

My body slowly but surely started rejecting foods one at a time, even the organic ones. My food would just come right back up, and more symptoms would accompany: horrible GI (gastrointestinal) pain and swelling, facial numbness, hives, dizziness and faintness, brain fog and confusion, heart palpations, facial and throat swelling, swelling in different organs, lethargy, weakness, joint and bone pains, the D word that no one likes to talk about, extreme tremors, sweating, nausea, and other symptoms I'm sure I've forgotten about. You could kind of relate it to the worst food poisoning you have ever experienced times ten and then just add in all the other symptoms that I mentioned on top of that, and you may have a clearer picture of how horrible these reactions were.

During this time, I experienced multiple reactions that nearly landed me in the hospital as well as reactions that did. I was also suffering from so much GI pain that my gyn sent me to a GI specialist for a colonoscopy to check if the pain was from endometriosis (because I suffer from severe widespread endometriosis), but they found nothing abnormal at the time.

So, my doctor sent me to another allergist to see if he could figure something out because she had personally never seen anything like what I was going through. She also prescribed a new medication for me to try and ordered more blood work. When the labs came back, it showed that I had high thyroid antibodies, I was anemic, and I had a positive ANA, but this still didn't give insight as to what was going on. Because the thyroid antibodies were high, she sent a referral to an endocrinologist just in case the issue was stemming from that end.

The first appointment to come was with the endocrinologist. He came in and said that my antibodies were high, but all other thyroid functions were normal, and he felt comfortable in saying that whatever was happening wasn't because of the thyroid. He said that he wished he could help me, but he had seen nothing like what I was experiencing before, and his recommendation would be to see an allergist.

The second appointment was with the new allergist. As soon as I walked through his doors, I experienced an allergic reaction, and the nurses took me straight into the room. The doctor came in; he was very nice and said he wanted to run some more blood work. The blood work came back and showed that I tested positive for Alpha-gal syndrome. I asked what that was, and he explained that it is an allergy to red meat caused by a tick bite. This meant I needed to keep all red meat out of my diet. He also prescribed a new medication to try. So, I left the office with a little more hope in that we had found the answer as to what was going on.

I had never heard of Alpha-gal syndrome before, so I decided to read up a little more on this issue. I learned that Alpha-gal syndrome was a recently identified food allergy and that many doctors have never even heard of this illness.

Alpha-gal syndrome is shown to happen when the Lone Star tick bites a person and transmits a sugar molecule called "Alpha-gal" into his or her body. When this happens, it can trigger an immune reaction that can later cause mild to severe allergic reactions when that person encounters red meat, milk and mammalian byproducts, and unfortunately there is no cure. After learning a bit about Alpha-gal syndrome, I thought, *This is it. This is the break we have been waiting for.*

You see, I ate red meat mostly every day, I drank a creamy hot chocolate mocha every morning and afternoon, and I absolutely loved smothering my food in cheese. So, removing these things from my diet would surely help, but it was so hard to give up steak, tacos and hamburgers—honestly it still is. I had been taking the medications that the doctors had recently prescribed, but soon the side effects or reactions to the medications started outweighing the benefits. It turns out that a lot of medications contain a mammalian byproduct in the ingredients, and because of the

Alpha-gal syndrome, my body was not tolerating the medication.

Months had gone by, and I had cut out all items that could cause an Alpha-gal reaction, but I was still experiencing crazy symptoms, and my body started rejecting foods that had absolutely no mammalian byproducts in it. Additionally, my body became extremely reactive to chemicals, scents, cigarette smoke, and fumes from cooking. I decided to make another appointment with the allergist who had discovered the Alpha-gal allergy, but this time I prepared for the appointment by purchasing a very expensive top-brand allergy mask. That way, when I went into his office, I wouldn't go into an allergic reaction from the cleaning supplies they used in his building.

The morning of the appointment came, and I was ready. My husband helped me put the mask on properly, and we went in for the appointment. Within ten seconds of entering the building, my body experienced an allergic reaction again. I couldn't believe it. You would think that a top-of-the-line allergy mask would have helped. The nurses took me right back once again, and the doctor came in; he assured me that an allergy mask would not work for me because my body was so sensitive, and the particles in the air that I was reacting to were too small for the masks to filter out. We talked about everything I was going through and how I was still reacting and losing foods. Unfortunately, I had to hear the "wish I could help" speech, "but I don't know what to do." I do admire when doctors admit they don't know how to help and encourage you to find someone who would. So, he recommended that I see another GI specialist.

I had already had multiple visits with my doctor and traveled around the state, being seen by two allergists, an endocrinologist, a GI specialist, a rheumatologist and a gyn, and now I had another appointment with a new GI specialist. The GI specialist was a very unusual man but very knowledgeable in his field. During the appointment he mentioned wanting to check for mitral valve prolapse and do an endoscopy and a colonoscopy, but I could not tolerate the prep, so we could not do the colonoscopy.

The time arrived to drive to Birmingham in the early morning hours for the endoscopy procedure. Arriving early meant we had a good amount of time to go over things with the anesthesiologist. She decided that we needed to take precautions and administer medication without lidocaine and that she would stay in the room herself since it was so risky. I remember as soon as they started administering the medication, red lines appeared on my arm where the medication was flowing through the veins. It was such an intense, searing pain that I felt as if I were burning in a fiery furnace. The last thing I remember was the nurses holding me down, telling me it would all be over soon.

Next thing I know, I was coming to in recovery. It was very hard to open my eyes, but I could hear Christian music playing in the background and thought to myself, *Am I in heaven?* When I was able to open my eyes, I could see nurses busily running around. Then I heard the hospital speaker come on for a time of prayer. I remember thinking how amazing it was to wake up from something so scary and hear the peacefulness that surrounded me. I made sure to tell the nurse how just awesome it was, and she laughed because the effects from the medication were still taking a toll on me. The doctor said that the endoscopy looked good but that I did have a hiatal hernia, which was likely because of the stress of my body rejecting foods, and that the other test he ran showed mitral valve prolapse. He said he was confident in saying that I was experiencing something called dysautonomia, which is a condition in which the autonomic nervous system doesn't work properly.

Although the endoscopy didn't give us any information at the time, the biopsies that the doctor took would later provide important information. But at the moment we still didn't have any answers. We were back where we started, and I was steadily losing foods and experiencing weird symptoms, such as dizziness, faintness, rashes and hives just from attending a church service or simply walking into a store. It was like my body was turning completely against anything that I tried to do. I loved attending Sunday worship and enjoying the simple freedom of going into a store to get a small cup of coffee with a friend; I loved getting my hair done and wearing makeup, but all the little things that I took for granted slowly faded away.

Chapter 3

Where Are You Now?

 As time went on and things became worse, I questioned God. I didn't understand why this was happening to me and why He would allow this to continue, but even though I didn't understand why I was having to go through so much suffering, I still chose to put my trust in Him because He promised that He would never leave or forsake me. During this raging storm that was ripping through my life, that was a promise I was holding onto. Knowing that He was my strength in the storm gave me hope to not give up.

I still didn't understand though. I mean, I had given my life to Christ, was serving in the ministry at the time and fully believed in the healing power of Christ, as I had seen His power firsthand and still believed that He could heal. I prayed multiple times a day, spent alone time in worship every chance I got and just tried to show the love of Christ in my everyday life, but no matter how much good I did, I was just becoming sicker and sicker. I felt so alone, and I could feel that death was close. At one point, I actually started to fear praying because it seemed that the more I prayed, the worse things would get. I began to question God. I asked Him where He was at. Why had He not healed me yet? What did I do to deserve this?

I mean, so many people out there were living so much worse than I was. Don't get me wrong; I am far from perfect, but their lives were going great and they were healthy. I remember just crying every day because I didn't foresee this for myself. When I had envisioned my future, I had seen so many open doors into different areas of the ministry that I wanted to experience. I never foresaw contracting an illness that would take away a large portion of those dreams from me, much less the simple freedom of attending a church service. You would think that if God had called you into the ministry, He would make a way for you to be a part of a ministry, right? Even though I had all of these thoughts, all I could do was hang onto Him, because even in life or death and health and sickness, He is still the King of Kings. Just as Paul said, "For to me to live is Christ and to die is gain," I knew the moment I breathed my last breath I would see my Beloved's face and all the suffering would end.

One of my favorite historical events in Jesus's life that always seemed to stir up inside of me when I began to question my suffering is the time when Jesus was crossing the Sea of Galilee.

"And there arose a great storm of wind, and the waves beat into the ship, so that it was now full... And He arose, and rebuked the wind and said unto the sea, Peace, be still. And the wind ceased, and there was a great calm" (Mark 4:37,39) TMB.

What's so inspiring to me about this occasion is that Jesus was on a path that would bring to pass one of His most astonishing miracles to date: casting a multitude of demons out of a man that was well-known and very much feared throughout the whole territory.

While on this path, Jesus and His disciples found themselves in the middle of an out-of-the-blue, epically ferocious windstorm that could have easily overturned their ship.

Could it have been that during this moment in time, Satan knew what was about to transpire and wanted to keep it from happening? If Jesus was to continue on His current course, then He would eventually reach the possessed man, freeing him from all demonic bondage, resulting in Satan losing one of his most valuable assets in the area.

Without thinking twice, Jesus stood up to the plate and took charge over the entire situation, commanding the winds to cease and they did!

This event encourages me and helps to remind me that anytime we are doing something that will advance the

25

Kingdom of God, whether it be in our own lives or the lives of others, different types of attacks may come upon us. It's not that we have done something wrong and are being punished but that we are actually doing something right. When these attacks come we have to learn to rely on God, to trust that He can see the bigger picture and to stand firm in the authority that Christ has given us over our situations.

Then, when the storms are raging, we can remember that even during the most violent of storms, Jesus is still the Lord, and He can calm all the wind and the waves that life may throw at us. He is right there beside us, fighting for us, even during the times when we think and feel like He isn't near us. He truly is right there, and believe me, I spent a lot of lonely nights in a hospital bed asking why He felt so far away. Little did I know He was right there in that hospital room with me. He never left me, and I can clearly see that now, even though I couldn't then.

The thing I love about this historical event is the fact that during this vicious storm, Jesus was actually sleeping, and the disciples rushed over to wake Him up, asking Him, "Teacher, do you not care if we drown?" and after Jesus woke up and calmed the storm, He asked them, "Why are you afraid? Do you have no faith?"

Even the disciples, the men who spent their days in the very presence of Jesus, still got scared and asked Jesus if He cared.

Chapter 4

RMSF, How Are You Alive?

As my symptoms began to drastically progress, my aunt who was also my nurse at the time ran a bunch of blood work, and since she had recently tested positive for Rocky Mountain spotted fever, she tested me for the disease as well. To our surprise, it came back positive! I had never heard of Rocky Mountain spotted fever before, but after learning that a tick bite caused this disease (and since I had already been diagnosed with Alpha-gal syndrome), I wondered how this could have possibly been missed. I mean, you would assume that if someone tested positive for one tick-borne illness the doctor would check for other tick-borne illnesses and coinfections, right? Unfortunately, that's not the case due to a lack of education on tick-borne illnesses in the medical community. In fact, most people with tick-borne illnesses go undiagnosed and misdiagnosed for years before finding out what is truly wrong with them, which is a very sad fact.

So, what exactly is Rocky Mountain spotted fever (RMSF)? It is actually one of the deadliest tick-borne diseases in the world, killing as many as 10% of people who have been infected by it. It is a bacterial infection (Rickettsia rickettsii) that is spread by the bite from an infected tick or being exposed to infected material from a crushed tick (although rarer) and is most commonly found in the southeastern United States, Canada, Mexico, Central America and South America. Once the bacterium is introduced to the body, it begins to spread through your bloodstream or lymphatic vessels and starts reproducing and causing damage inside living cells.

There are three commonly known types of ticks that carry Rickettsia rickettsii:

- The American dog tick (Dermacentor variabilis)
- The Rocky Mountain wood tick (Dermacentor andersoni)
- The brown dog tick (Rhipicephalus sanguineus)

Symptoms of Rocky Mountain spotted fever include:

- A distinctive rash that typically occurs after a fever
- Sensitivity to light
- Fever
- Headache
- Nausea and/or vomiting
- Stomach pains
- Muscle pains
- Lack of appetite

- Chills
- Joint pains

As I was researching and learning all of this new information, I realized that I had never had a major fever or experienced a rash like most people do who have the disease. I could not help but wonder just how long my body had been fighting this disease on its own and if that had been the cause for all the crazy, unimaginable things that I was going through. I learned that Rocky Mountain spotted fever can cause long-term effects and damage if it is not caught and treated properly, which in my case it was not. It also turns out that 10-15% of patients never develop a rash.

The doctor wrote a prescription for an antibiotic called doxycycline for me to start and wanted me to take it for fourteen days. Once we arrived at the pharmacy, the pharmacist informed us that the strength of the prescription she ordered contained red dye in it, which would cause an anaphylactic reaction if I was to take it, but she said a lower milligram they offered did not contain the red dye and that I would just have to take double the number of pills. We agreed, and she filled the medication, which meant I was to take ten pills a day of doxycycline.

I started taking the medication the very next day, and I immediately noticed its negative effect on me, but I tried to push through it. After a couple of days of taking the doxycycline, the symptoms became too much for me to handle—my GI system had become inflamed, and every time I attempted to take the doxycycline, my body started rejecting it and vomiting it back up—so at this point, I decided I could no longer put myself through this torment and stopped the doxycycline. I let my doctor know that my body was not handling the doxy, but at this point she did not offer any other treatment options. It turned out that the doxycycline pill contained mammalian byproducts, which caused my body to react because of the Alpha-gal syndrome, and I was attempting to force myself to take ten pills of this medication a day instead of two, so it's no wonder why my body rejected it.

A few months passed, and I was still going downhill, so my doctor's office ran more blood work, which also included another Rocky Mountain spotted fever test. This time the test came back a little higher. They waited and retested again a couple of months later, and the result still came back high. The doctor's office later received a call from the CDC that week concerning all of my test results regarding Rocky Mountain spotted fever. The CDC informed the doctor's office that I needed a referral to an infectious disease specialist to receive proper treatment, and they agreed. My doctor's office set up an appointment with an infectious disease specialist in Birmingham. At this point we were hopeful that this new doctor would be able to provide answers and provide a treatment so that I could get back to my normal, happy, busy life that I absolutely missed living.

The day of the appointment arrived. I remember taking the time to prepare a detailed list of everything I was going through and all the questions that I had to ask him, and then the moment of truth came. The doctor entered the room and right off the bat had a smug look, but I ignored it, introduced myself and started telling him why I was there. After I finished talking, he looked at me and said, "I don't care what the test results say, we do not have Rocky Mountain spotted fever or Lyme disease in Alabama."

Baffled by this, I told him that the CDC had sent me to him and said that I needed proper treatment for tick-borne illnesses, to which he replied while laughing, "I saw where the CDC requested you be seen, and the first thing I am going to do when I leave this room is call and give them a piece of my mind. We do not have Rocky Mountain spotted fever here, so they should have never sent you." He then asked, "Have you lived in or visited any other states?"

I replied, "Yes sir, Georgia, Tennessee, Pennsylvania, Oklahoma, West Virginia, Florida, Louisiana and a few other states I have visited," and his reply was "Those states don't have Rocky Mountain spotted fever either." at this point the appointment was over and our little bubble of hope was popped yet again. We were back where we started.

At this point I was losing hope in the medical community. No one knew what was going on. Doctors were just passing me back and forth, some showing compassion and really wanting to help but acknowledging that it was over their heads, while others just looked at me like I was crazy and then tried to prescribe a medication for anxiety which contained the same ingredients that they had just seen I was allergic too!

I fully believe that doctors should know what they are prescribing to their patients before giving it to them, don't you? For example, if the doctor has enough sense to check your blood work for red dye allergies, then you would think that he should have the knowledge not to prescribe a pill that has red dye in it if you are allergic to it, correct? Because what happens if that patient just puts her trust in her doctor and takes the medication as prescribed and then has an allergic reaction to the medication because of the red dye? Whose fault would it have been—the professionals who spent years in school or the patient who is blindly putting her trust in her medical provider like she has been told to do? This happened to me several times with the medications being prescribed containing mammalian byproducts, leading to a reaction.

I personally believe that Alpha-gal syndrome should be taken just as seriously as a shellfish or peanut allergy. There should be warning labels on all products just as there are for a peanut allergy, even if it's something simple that says "this item may contain animal byproducts." I for one can say without a shadow of a doubt that a label like this would save a lot of people from experiencing allergic reactions, because most of the time ingredient lists will say "natural flavors," but in all actuality the natural flavor is really beef broth.

Someone new to Alpha-gal syndrome would have no clue about this; they would just be looking for the word "beef," not "natural flavorings." This is a lesson I had to learn the hard way. I eventually started breaking every ingredient down because unfortunately animal byproducts can be listed under many different names. A label that would warn of animal byproducts would truly help children such as my son who may not comprehend what all ingredients to look out for, but they would understand to watch out for a warning label.

I also strongly believe that all doctors should be aware and informed of the high risk of an allergic response to vaccines in children and adults with Alpha-gal syndrome, as most vaccines contain animal byproducts. To take it a little further, due to the increasing rates of Alpha-gal syndrome, I believe that we should incorporate the Alpha-Gal Panel testing into our children's yearly schedule prior to receiving vaccinations. I've personally had firsthand experience with vaccine reactions because of this issue, and I can tell you it's not pretty and it's very scary to have to deal with it, especially when it could have been prevented had the doctors had the appropriate knowledge on the subject. And while we're at it, let's give some funding toward having vaccine safety studies done.

I went online to try to find others who had been diagnosed with alpha-gal syndrome and Rocky Mountain spotted fever to see if there was anyone else who was experiencing what I was going through, and that's when I found support groups on Facebook. I asked to join the few groups I found and read through the content but didn't see anyone who was experiencing the extremity of things like I was, so I decided to make a post on the groups, asking for advice. This turned out to be extremely helpful as a lot of people contacted me, asking if I had been tested for a condition called mast cell activation syndrome. I told them that I had not been checked for it, nor had it been mentioned.

Chapter 5

What is Mast Cell Activation Syndrome?

After reaching out to the Facebook support groups and being encouraged to look into something called "mast cell activation syndrome," I took to the internet and started reading any and all medical articles I could find on the subject, and I was so surprised because it was describing everything I was going through to a T! So, what exactly is a mast cell, and what the heck is mast cell activation syndrome?

Well, to start with, a mast cell is a type of immune cell—kind of like your body's own little soldier that tries to protect you by detecting and responding to foreign substances. They can be found throughout the body, particularly under the skin, in the gastrointestinal tract, surrounding lymph vessels and bloods vessels, in nerves and in the lungs. They perform a significant job in anaphylaxis and help guard against pathogens. When a mast cell is triggered and activated, it can release more than 200 chemical meditators, which leads to symptoms. Many things can activate a mast cell, such as environmental toxins, viruses, parasites, mold toxicity and tick-borne diseases.

Wait, what? Tick-borne illnesses can cause a mast cell to become active? The answer, to my surprise, was yes! This is because our mast cells are a part of our bodies' defense system, and when a tick-borne illness, such as Rocky Mountain spotted fever, Alpha-gal syndrome, Lyme disease and/or coinfections, are introduced to our bodies, our mast cells recognize it as a foreign invader and attack it, releasing many chemical mediators that it is prepacked with to try to defeat the said pathogen. In my case, due to the tick-borne illnesses going undiagnosed and untreated for so long, my body tried to rise up and defeat these illnesses on its own, and it has not stopped waging war since mistaking foods, medications, chemicals, perfumes, cigarette smoke, herbicides, pesticides, city water, heat/cold and even large amounts of sunshine as invaders.

Now that we know what a mast cell is, what is mast cell activation syndrome?

Mast cell activation syndrome (MCAS) is a recently identified immune condition where a patient's mast cells release chemical mediators too frequently and too often, which causes the patient to experience repeated episodes of anaphylactic symptoms.

According to Dr. Denise Clark, (2018) Mast Cell and Tick-Borne Disease Specialist:

Symptoms of MCAS can be similar to many other diseases, which makes it difficult to diagnose. The most common symptom is rapid onset after eating of flushing, palpitations, itching, tongue swelling, wheezing, gas, bloating, nausea, vomiting, abdominal pain, and dizziness. Research indicates that it is an under-recognized contributor to neurologic and psychiatric symptoms as well as multiple chemical sensitivities. A key to diagnosis is if water or food, any food, sets off a reaction and in 3-5 minutes reproducible symptoms occur. (para. 3)

Other symptoms of mast cell activation syndrome can include:

- Neurological issues, such as headache, brain fog, cognitive dysfunction, anxiety, depression
- Nasal itching and congestion, throat itching and swelling, wheezing and shortness of breath, difficulty taking deep breaths
- Diarrhea, vomiting, nausea, abdominal pain, bloating, GERD, GI inflammation
- Bone/muscle pain, osteopenia, osteoporosis
- Bladder irritability, frequent voiding

- Flushing of the skin (face/neck/chest), hives, skin irritations, rashes and itching with or without hives
- Lightheadedness, fainting, rapid heart rate, chest pain, low blood pressure, high blood pressure
- Uterine cramps, heavy and painful periods, bleeding and endometriosis
- Anaphylaxis, angioedema (swelling)
- Malnutrition and dehydration
- Intolerance of heat or cold
- Potential swelling in any part of the body
- Environmental allergies, medication and chemical sensitivities
- Vision disturbances
- Difficulty swallowing
- Poor wound healing
- Asthma
- Hair thinning and loss
- Fatigue, insomnia
- Tremors
- Excessive sweating
- Sores in the mouth
- Easy bleeding and bruising
- Enlargement and tender lymph nodes

Wow, that's a lot of symptoms. But even after reading the list, most people will never comprehend what it's like to actually live with this illness. Just to put it in perspective, many of us are familiar with the symptoms of chemotherapy, and if you're like me, your heart is filled with compassion toward someone going through that battle because it's a major life-changing life-or-death event. I have seen patients who had previously battled cancer and won (thank God) but were now living with mast cell activation syndrome stemming from tick-borne disease, and according to their personal experiences, living with the everyday symptoms of mast cell activation syndrome was worse than going through the symptoms of chemotherapy. This should give us a clear picture that living with mast cell activation syndrome is not a minor battle that can be overlooked or worked through. This is a life-changing life-or-death event.

Dr. Afrin, one of the leading mast cell activation syndrome experts in the nation, said, "It's hard to imagine a disease more complex than mast cell activation syndrome."

I learned that patients who suffer from mast cell activation syndrome can have an allergic response to things such as:

- Food and beverages, including bottled and city water

- Pharmaceutical drugs and contrast dyes
- Exercise
- Natural and chemical odors, including cigarette smoke, pesticides, herbicides, perfumes/scents and even fumes from cooking foods
- Venom from a bee, wasp, spider, fire ant, snake, or jelly fish, and bites from a mosquito or flea
- Viral, bacterial and fungal infections
- Vibrations, friction or mechanical irritation to skin
- Pain
- Sun/sunlight
- Hot or cold temperatures
- Environmental pollution and mold exposure
- Hormonal fluctuations
- Additives in foods and medications

After doing a lot of research regarding how this disease affects patients and how each patient can react or respond to things so differently—along with the fact that most doctors have never heard of this syndrome, much less know how to test for it or treat it properly—I have to completely agree with Dr. Afrin's statement.

After learning all of this new information, I started forwarding some of the medical research articles on mast cell activation syndrome to my nurse, who shared it with my doctor, who agreed that I needed to be tested for this condition. But mast cell activation syndrome can be difficult to diagnose and is often missed because of its complexity and the fact that standard testing may reveal nothing abnormal at the time As of right now, there is no standard diagnosing protocol set for MCAS, but when it comes to diagnosing, the doctor will look at:

1. Clinical presentation (does the patient's history and symptoms line up with mast cell activation syndrome?)
2. Elevated biopsies or laboratory evidence of mast cell activation
3. Ruling out all other possible diseases

We decided to schedule an appointment with an allergist as well as reach back out to the gastrologist who had previously done the upper endoscopy and taken multiple biopsies, hoping that maybe the hospital lab might have the biopsies still there. If so, those biopsies could be tested, keeping me from having to go through another procedure to collect new biopsies. The gastrologist said he had never heard of mast cell activation syndrome but would look into it and order the proper test needed. Two weeks had gone by, and I received a letter in the mail from the GI specialist. It was the test results from the biopsies he had ordered.

The results showed increased mast cells (CD117 staining) in both my stomach and duodenum. I forwarded these results to my primary doctor and then went to talk with the allergist who had some knowledge on mast cell activation syndrome. He prescribed compounded Benadryl and cromolyn sodium, which is a mast cell stabilizing medication, and gave me the information to a mast cell activation syndrome specialist out of New York to schedule an appointment with. After I met certain criteria, my doctors officially diagnosed me with mast cell activation syndrome brought on by the tick-borne illnesses going untreated.

We found a compounding pharmacy in town that agreed to provide the straight cromolyn and Benadryl powder to mix in my well water at home. That way, there would be no fillers or additives that could cause me to react. I was a little nervous and excited at the same time about this new treatment. I mean, this could possibly help give me a somewhat normal life again! The doctor advised that I start taking little amounts at a time and work my way up, which was also the advice of other mast cell patients. I also heard a lot of people say that with this medication, symptoms may get worse before they get better and to just push on through it.

Well, day one was great, and day two was even better! I felt amazing. I was even able to get up to clean the house—something which, at that point in time, I had not had the strength to do. A few more days went by, and everything was going great until the second week hit. The medication started having time to build up in my system, and my body started fighting against it. It started out with a small lump on one side of my throat that started getting larger and more painful day by day. Then my face and chest broke out in acne like blisters, and my eyes and tongue swelled. I took the Benadryl as prescribed, but it didn't faze my symptoms. My husband called the allergist, who wanted him to administer an EpiPen, but at the time only half of my throat was swollen, and even though I couldn't swallow I was scared at what the Epi might do because I had never used it before, so as long as I could breathe, I wouldn't let him administer it. It took two weeks to recover from that reaction, and it went away gradually just as it had come on and was one of the worst cases of throat swelling, I had experienced up to that point. I decided there was no way I was trying that treatment option again, but it did turn out that I tolerated the compounded Benadryl.

Although we had gotten some answers regarding MCAS, my local doctors didn't know what to do except try to get me to see a mast cell specialist as quickly as possible, which was not an easy task because there are very few mast cell specialists in the entire nation, and they all seemed to be across country.

Chapter 6

Have a Seat

A few months passed, and then the unexpected happened. I started having pains in the joints of my feet, especially my big toe joints. It felt as if someone were slicing me open from the inside out. Then I started getting pains down deep in my bones, and next thing I knew I began to lose feeling deep inside my joints. They began to turn a deep dark purple. Then I began to lose the ability to move my joints, and extreme neuropathy started to set in—a never-ending, unimaginable burning as if my skin were melting off of my body that began in my feet, working its way up my legs. The pain was so unbearable that even the slightest breeze of air would send me into excruciating pain and tears. I couldn't even bear to cover my lower extremities with a light sheet, and we didn't dare try to bathe them because as soon as anything touched my skin, the burning feeling would intensify until I became so nauseated and in and out of reality that I would hear crying only to realize it was me crying out in pain. I lost my ability to walk. I could not even stretch my legs out straight anymore or wiggle my toes, and I was in such constant pain that I was only sleeping one hour a day in a twenty-four-hour period, and the only reason that I slept that hour is because my body would just black out, and then I would come back to.

Losing the simple freedom of walking really took its toll on me. I can recall, before getting my wheelchair, lying on a pallet in the living room floor while no one was home. It was snowing outside, and I really just wanted to feel the snow on my skin. I decided that I would try to make it to the front door, but to do that I had to pull myself across the floor like a lame animal. It was very difficult, but I was finally able to reach the doorknob and use enough strength to open it and lie in the doorway with my hand outside in the snow.

Before being bitten by a tick, I was extremely active, very outspoken and full of life. Any time I walked into a room people would take notice, offering up a kind smile while they went about their day, but that all changed once I became wheelchair-bound. I am not sure what changed exactly, but when I entered the room, no one seemed to notice I was even there. Everyone would go about their day as if I were completely invisible, and this really bothered me because it was a complete change for me—a part of the world that I hadn't experienced or even thought about before.

Growing up in the South, I was familiar with people greeting others with smiles as part of that sweet southern charm, but instead of experiencing that, I was now being greeted by people who were obviously trying to not make eye contact, as if something was wrong with me and I was being shunned, or they would just stare.

I tried not to let it bother me even though deep down it hurt my feelings and self-esteem, but I realized that I was looking at it from the wrong perspective. I thought to myself that maybe it wasn't that I was invisible but rather that a large majority of society simply might not know what to do when they encounter someone who cannot walk and needs the help of a wheelchair. Because of that, I couldn't be mad or let that situation make me bitter because it could just as easily have been me unknowingly reacting the same way if put in the same situation, not knowing what I know now. I had to learn to roll out of my comfort zone and keep rolling past all of the stares, offering a gentle smile even when others wouldn't.

This experience taught me personally how to react when I am in that situation. I now know from personal experience that a mere smile can change someone's entire day—and, who knows, maybe even someone's life. People appreciate knowing that they are seen and are not invisible or any less of a person just because they have a disability that they cannot help. I can sincerely say that this ordeal completely changed the way I view life, and I will remember it for an eternity.

Chapter 7

Near Death

At this point things were becoming very scary. I had lost all of my foods and was surviving only on certain brands of organic diced tomatoes, flour, blueberries and maple syrup. It was very disgusting to eat diced tomatoes and noodles made from flour and water three times a day every day with no salt or flavor, but I had to push through if I wanted to survive.

My husband was not only having to make fresh handmade flour noodles every day, bless his heart, but he was also having to drive an hour a day just to fill up a glass gallon jar of well water from his dad's house because it was the only thing I could drink, as I had started reacting to city and bottled water. When I first started reacting to water, we were so confused. I had already lost everything ranging from juices to dairy, and now water! We all need water to survive. This made absolutely no sense. We discovered that it was not the water itself I was reacting to but rather the toxic chemicals like PFAS, which is a group of more than 5,000 toxic chemicals that are found in our city and bottled water supplies. Exposure to these chemicals has been linked to:

- Cancers and tumors
- Suppression of the immune system
- Hormonal disruption of the thyroid
- High cholesterol levels
- Atopic dermatitis

PFAS can build up in our bodies and can be found in breast milk, blood, umbilical cord blood and urine. PFAS may also be linked to:

- Lowering the chance of becoming pregnant
- Developmental effects in infants
- Low birth weight

Unfortunately, PFAS is not the only toxic contaminates found in our water supplies. We also must watch out for things like disinfectant byproducts, which have been linked to cancer and reproductive issues along with developmental issues. Pesticides and herbicides have also been found in city and bottled water.

And if my body's reaction to water wasn't bad enough, I also tried every brand of organic or all-natural vitamins that I could find in the health food store but still could not get my body to accept them. My strength was fading away with every new day to the point that I even sucked up the courage to cut off and donate my beautiful long hair because I could not find the strength to lift the brush up to brush it, not to mention the fact that my hair was falling out in large masses. I absolutely loved my waist-length hair—it made me feel safe—and chopping it off was absolutely heartbreaking.

During this time, my husband had to start staying home as I needed a caregiver 24/7. We reached out to the mast cell specialist in New York to schedule an appointment and get the information on what it would cost to be seen. The office informed us that the doctor was not accepting new patients at the moment but would be at the beginning of the new year, which was around seven months or so away, and stated that I could be put at the top of the waiting list to be seen since my situation was more urgent. They informed us the first visit was $2,000 as well as the follow-up visit, totaling $4,000 for the first two initial visits.

My insurance did not cover a penny of it, not to mention the additional upfront cost of all the medical tests the doctor would need to order, treatment costs and travel expenses to stay in New York for one to two weeks, which all added up fast. At that moment I knew there was no way that I was going to be able to cover all of this myself with my husband having to stop working to be able to take care of me. I felt so helpless, but my grandma and family encouraged me not to give up because God had a plan for my life, and He would provide a way. So we went ahead and gave the office permission to add me to the waiting list with the hopes that by the time they called to schedule the appointment, we would have the funds saved up.

I called my neurologist, whom I had previously seen for the seizure like activity that I was experiencing during or after allergic reactions. I told the office what was going on, and they scheduled an appointment to see me right away. This was terrifying to me. Why had I suddenly lost my ability to walk, and why did my skin feel like it was melting off of my body?

The neurologist's office said to be there early in the morning; they would work me in because otherwise he was booked up for weeks. Early that next morning, my husband carried me to the truck and put me in the front seat, and my son sat in the back seat. My husband had previously loaded up my electric wheelchair the night before, so we were all set to go.

We were almost to the neurologist's office when suddenly a vehicle two cars ahead of us slammed on their brakes, causing the car in front of us to rear-end them and us to rear-end the car in front of us. The car that initially slammed on their brakes drove off, leaving the scene. The cops arrived to take an accident report, which was putting us behind. I instantly called the neurologist's office and told them what had happened. They explained that since I was fifteen minutes late, the doctor couldn't see me, and it would be a few weeks before he could. At this point I was crushed and started crying uncontrollably. People at the scene took notice, but I just couldn't help it. I could not take it anymore. I was experiencing such an intense burning pain that I honestly imagined it was what the deepest parts of hell felt like.

The neurologist's office encouraged me to go to the emergency room. However, emergency rooms are a dangerous place for someone with mast cell activation syndrome because of exposures not only to chemicals, perfumes and smokers but also to germs that can cause sicknesses. Even something as simple as the common cold can greatly affect someone with mast cell activation syndrome much more than a normal healthy person. All in all, emergency rooms were my last resort, but I knew I was about to die. I could feel it in my soul.

The paramedics arrived to take me to the local emergency room in Tuscaloosa, and the plan was to be put in a room or area away from the waiting room and others, since it posed such an enormous risk. I typically never arrived at the hospital by myself, because during reactions I could not speak up for myself, but on this day my husband had to drive behind the ambulance instead of riding with me.

I arrived at the hospital in the ambulance; they took me in and put me in a wheelchair, but this wheelchair wasn't a normal wheelchair. All of the wheels were small, meaning this type of wheelchair was meant for someone who had function of the lower limbs, which I didn't. They then started pushing me into the ER waiting room that was packed full of people, where I instantly started reacting. My whole chest broke out in a solid rash, burning hot, and I started vomiting. I told them, "You cannot leave me in here. I am reacting to something, and I need you to push the wheelchair outside."

They said they could not do that; I would have to talk with the nurse at the ER desk. At this point she saw the commotion and walked over. I explained to her that I had mast cell activation syndrome and that I was reacting to something in the ER and needed to be pushed out of there. She replied rudely that she had never heard of mast cell activation syndrome before and proceeded to shove—and I mean shove—a paper face mask on my face and then squeezed it painfully on my nose. If this woman would have tried to do this to me when I could have defended myself, she wouldn't have succeeded in putting her hands on me, but I was weak, in a reaction and didn't have control of my lower limbs. I was helpless.

I took out my phone and called my nurse, crying hysterically and telling her what had just happened and that

I was in the ER and staff was refusing to push me outside. At that point my husband came through the ER doors, saw what was happening and started demanding to see someone because "there should be hospital protocols in place for patients with immune disorders." Within moments they had me in triage and in a room.

The hospital doctor finally came in and said that all the tests they ran came back great and everything was normal. I asked him about vitamin levels, and he said that they were all normal as well, and he didn't know why I lost the ability to function in the lower part of my body or why I was experiencing extreme burning neuropathy. After begging him, he agreed to admit me in the hospital to run a few more tests, but he encouraged me to seek out a nutritionist. They admitted me to the hospital and ran more blood work; the doctor came in the next morning and said that my potassium was a little low and that I should try some B12 shots, but he had no clue what was going on, so they released me from the hospital that day.

Chapter 8

Malnutrition and Dehydration

We were in complete disbelief that I was being let go from the hospital, with no explanation as to why certain things were happening in my body. We took the B12 prescription that the hospital doctor had prescribed and had it filled at the compounding pharmacy. From there we headed to my hometown doctor's office for them to show us how to properly give a shot at home since I was now prescribed a shot daily for a certain period of time.

When we got to the office, my husband lifted me into his arms and gently set me into the wheelchair, and we headed toward the back entrance of the office, as the nurse would meet us there to avoid risking exposure to something in the main office. The back door swung open, and my aunt stepped out. I could see the look of concern on her face when she saw me, as if she was scared but wanted to put on a brave face for me. She knew I was bad, but I don't think she realized just how bad. It was not too terribly long after I left the office that I received a call from my aunt; she had found a nutritionist in Birmingham, AL. When the doctor's office reached out to him and explained the situation and that they feared I wouldn't survive it much longer, he agreed to see me right away.

By this point every moment and every heartbeat was torture. The pain never ceased. I couldn't get out of bed, much less use the bathroom by myself. I was helpless, missing precious moments in my family's lives. At the time I couldn't eat anything but nasty diced tomatoes and noodles made from flour and water. I couldn't sleep but an hour a day because of the pain, and I began to just cry out to God because I felt so alone, so abandoned. Where was He? Where was my miracle? I didn't understand then and I honestly still don't now, but one thing is for certain: I will never let Him go even in the midst of the darkest night because I know He will always be there, and His light outshines even the darkest hour.

Between the burning torture and the lack of sleep, my mind became depressed, and all I could do was cry. I was holding onto hope that either Jesus was about to heal me or I was about to meet Him face to face. Either option sounded good to me at the time, but I just couldn't give up.

I wanted to see my son turn eleven; I wanted to be there when he met his first love, got married and created a family of his own. I wanted to one day have the experience of looking down into the eyes of my precious big-eyed grandchild, knowing that my love story helped to bring another amazing person into the world. I wanted to be there hand in hand with my husband and look back, knowing that we overcame and did all we had planned to do together. I just wanted to live; I didn't want to say goodbye. I didn't want my story to end there because I hadn't had enough time to fully live yet.

The time came for my husband to pack everything into the truck and take me to the nutritionist appointment. I remember the feeling of the cold, crisp air hitting my face as my husband carried me out of our house to the front seat of the truck. I was so weak and tired that I had contemplated not making the drive to Birmingham, because by this point my weight was down to around eighty-five pounds. I had lost a large majority of my body's muscle mass and had begun to look like someone you might have seen from pictures of the holocaust, and it became very obvious that I was losing this battle.

We arrived at the nutritionist's office. As my husband began pushing the wheelchair up to the receptionist's desk to sign in, I noticed that this office had very subtle pictures, magazines, books and inspirational quotes placed throughout the office on the subject of Jesus. This was different to me and not what I was used to seeing in all the other offices I had been in, and even though I feared what the doctor might say, I had a sense of peace come into my spirit, like God was saying, "I got you" and I was where I was supposed to be.

As I got closer to the counter, the receptionist stood up, and I could see her warm, welcoming smile. Once my husband signed me in, she told us that the doctor was not in the office yet, but she could tell that, just by looking at me, he was going to want to admit me into the hospital on the spot. So, she asked if it would be alright if she went ahead and called the hospital to arrange a room for me to be admitted.

Wait! What? That was not what I was expecting to hear. I mean, how would this even work? I had to be on a strict routine just to survive, a hospital setting had proven time and time again that it caused allergic reactions because of different triggers such as perfumes and disinfectants in the air, and the hospital could not provide my safe foods in a sterile environment. With those thoughts coming into my head as well as Christmas being right around the corner, I politely declined and told her I would like to hear what the doctor had to say first.

We ended up having to wait a few hours, but the doctor finally arrived. My husband rolled me into the exam room. The doctor was very nice, and he really listened. He then told me that he wanted to admit me into the hospital to receive nutrition through a PICC line. As he said this, the panic set in like it had when his receptionist mentioned it, and I think he could see the fear and hesitation in my eyes because he proceeded to try to calmly assure me that he felt I would not make it very long if I left his office that day.

He explained that I was extremely malnourished and dehydrated due to the mast cell activation syndrome and Alpha-gal syndrome, limiting what foods and liquids I could safely eat. He said that just as a car needs fuel to keep going, our bodies need the proper nutrition to continue working. He felt that my joints turning a dark purple and the loss of feeling in my feet and legs as well as the unbearable, torturous, extreme burning neuropathy and a few other symptoms I was experiencing was from my body basically eating itself to stay alive. My system had to take that nutrition from somewhere when it was not getting enough from my food intake, and because of this I was experiencing nerve damage.

I told him that all the other doctors tested my vitamin levels and said they were all normal. He then proceeded to tell me that when someone becomes as malnourished and dehydrated as I was, the blood work can come back showing false normal levels due to the fact that the body/fluid ratio levels were not correct because of the dehydration. To better help me understand what he meant, he told me to think of a can of frozen condensed orange juice; the juice is too strong on its own, so you have to mix it with water to dilute it down to the proper juice/water ratio for drinking. It was the same with the blood work; it was too condensed, giving off false normal results. But, in all reality, if I had the proper hydration and not been so dehydrated, the blood work would have shown the low vitamin levels because the blood they tested wouldn't have been so concentrated, so to say.

After talking with him a little while longer and him stressing his concern, we agreed to go ahead and let him admit me into the hospital. His receptionist came into the room and told us that the hospital had a room ready and that she would escort us over to be admitted through the ER and up into a room. I know I already said how scary this was for me, but this was very scary because I just knew it was this or death, and I was not even sure that I would be leaving that hospital alive.

After they settled me into a room, the doctor came in to go over what he wanted to do, and at that point he said that I needed rest before he could do anything. I was so sleep-deprived, and for the body to heal it needs rest, so he prescribed IV Benadryl every two hours along with Demerol. This was the first time in I don't know how long that I was able to fall asleep! Of course, the medications knocked me out, but it's what I needed. I could sleep for an hour and a half, and then I would be awakened by the excruciating, burning pain and would have to suffer until the next two-hour mark, where I received more Benadryl and pain medication. My husband and son were not able to stay up there with me that night because of multiple reasons:

1. I did not have safe food or water up there, so my husband would have to drive back and forth over an hour away to cook my food and fill up my water jug daily.

2. All of this, along with the out-of-pocket cost for compounded medications, left us without enough money to cover a hotel stay with enough food for them.

This was the first time I had ever been away from my son and my husband. Honestly, I don't think I can even recall a time where I have ever had to stay by myself before, so just being left alone was hard enough. My husband came up with the idea to call me right before they went to bed, leaving his phone on speaker call throughout the entire night. That way, I wouldn't feel so alone, and he would have the assurance that I was okay. Even though I had nurses coming in and out every hour or so, and even with my husband on the phone 24/7, I just could not shake the isolated feeling of the cold sterile hospital room.

Christmastime was just around the corner. Normally around this time of year I was used to a house filled with magical Christmas decor, presents overflowing under the tree, and being surrounded by my family and friends, enjoying our time together as we celebrated the birth of Jesus. Christmas has always been an enormous celebration to our family. My grandmother especially loved everything about Christmas, and all her Christmas spirit could turn even the coldest Grinch warm. She always made sure that everything was perfect and grand, which included her attempting to have the brightest decorated yard in the entire neighborhood, a table full of southern home cooking, and presents almost as high as her Christmas trees! Yes, you heard me correctly—she had multiple Christmas trees, an upside-down tree and an angel tree that she loved so much she kept them up year-round.

On Christmas Eve all of our family would return home together, cherishing the new memories that we were creating, and at the end of the day we would gather in a circle by the Christmas trees to pass around gifts, watching each other's face light up in glee when it was time to open our presents.

Christmas day morning was always a little more personal. The morning would normally start with our son pouncing on us while we were still asleep before the sun rose because of the inability to contain his excitement about the day and, of course, the gifts under the tree. We would hop out of bed and meet him in the living room, where he sat patiently waiting beside the pile of presents under the tree. But our tradition is a little different from others; instead of thanking Santa for the gifts, we always prayed together as a family, thanking God for blessing us with the funds to provide the gifts under the tree and giving thanks for the best gift of all—His son, Jesus.

I could close my eyes and melt away into these memories, but I would soon fade back into reality as soon as I opened my eyes. Instead of colorful tassels glimmering in the lights, I was surrounded by tubes and bland neutral-color walls, with a view overlooking a parking lot hours away from my family. Would I make it till Christmas, I wondered? I did not want to go home to heaven during the Christmas season because I did not want to ruin the magic of Christmas for my son, nor did I want it to serve as a reminder of him losing his mom.

I wondered how he was handling me not being at home and how Christmas morning would go. My family had already decided to cancel Christmas Eve plans until I could be there, and it wasn't but a day or so prior my son had crawled up into my hospital bed beside me, snuggled in and just started crying his eyes out while he held me. He wasn't ready to say goodbye to his mom. What ten-year-old would be? At that moment, I knew that even though my strength was rapidly fading away, I had to keep going. I could not bear the thought of leaving my baby in this big world without a momma. So, we held each other, let out all our tears, and prayed. It's not often I see my son break down, but I know that day God heard that baby's prayers.

Christmas morning came around. I woke up peering out of my window to watch the sun rise over the busy hospital roof and parking lot, but soon my hospital door burst open with my handsome husband and son walking in, both with glowing smiles upon their faces. Both of their arms were filled with miniature potted flowers of many different colors. "Merry Christmas!" they shouted as they came toward my bed. They set the flowers in the windowsill, and as my son climbed up in my bed to snuggle, still in his pajamas, my husband leaned in to plant a big warm loving kiss upon my forehead as he told me he would be right back. Our son's face was lit up with excitement, and he was so happy to be there with me to celebrate Christmas morning.

His dad walked back into the room, this time with a bag full of gifts. They sat in a circle around my bed. We prayed together, thanking God not only for His amazing Son and the gifts that He provided but also for allowing me to make one more Christmas memory, and at that moment it didn't matter where we were. We were together, and that was the only thing that mattered.

After a couple of days of receiving the IV fluids, Benadryl and pain medication, the doctor felt it was time to start IV vitamins, and at first it seemed to be going well as far as reactions went—nothing was swelling, and there were no hives. The doctor scheduled a physical therapist to come in and give an evaluation to see what she recommended for my lower extremities. When she came in, she had a goal of getting me to sit up in a bedside chair and straighten my legs. This was an extreme challenge for both of us, as she had to help lift me into the chair, where she propped up my legs and tried to straighten them. The pain just overtook me, and tears burst out of my eyes. I could do nothing but cry out in extreme pain. She said that was enough and put me back in bed. She then told me she was recommending physical therapy every day, and her recommendation to the doctor was to admit me into the hospital rehab for three months for physical therapy.

This shook me. Three months? After compiling what all was happening in reality, I realized this wasn't something that was going to go away overnight. This was a battle that was going to take months, if I could even make it that long. And would I ever even be able to walk again?

With the hospital unable to provide my food, my husband brought up a cooler to keep my food in and a hot plate to warm it so it wasn't freezing (after all, it was hard enough to eat nasty bitter diced tomatoes and flour noodles). Unfortunately, one of the nurses saw the hot plate and put in a complaint, as it was against the hospital's rules to have hot plates or electric burners in the rooms. After a few meetings with hospital staff and administrators, they agreed to let my husband heat up my food in the bathroom—yes, the bathroom, of all places—because it was the only safe place due to fire code, but I was just extremely grateful they allowed us to do this because without that, I wouldn't have had any type of food.

We noticed that I was having a harder time swallowing food or water, and it seemed as if my GI system was slowing down, and without access to my food, I was sure the loss of function I seemed to be experiencing would just become worse because even though I was starving to death, the diced tomatoes had to be doing something to keep me alive.

The nurses were genuinely nice, and the doctor himself went out of his way to be there to show he cared. I remember he would come in at night and just sit with me, sometimes for hours. We would talk about Jesus, and he would give me encouragement as well as make me feel not so alone. I'm not sure if he even realized it or not, but I needed those talks just as much as I needed nutrition because him being there and our talks were just another reminder that God was with me. When you're in such a dark place in life, as I was in at that moment, it was like breathing a breath of life into something that's hanging on by a thread, and during that time I was just hanging by a thread. I had already begun to make plans for my own funeral as well as making goodbye videos.

My doctor's original plan was to have a PICC line placed in my arm, and he scheduled to have the PICC line nurse come in to go over the procedure before they scheduled it. But the unexpected happened—my IV site became swollen, red and very painful. I called the nurse in, and she removed it, placed the IV in another location, and let the doctor know what had happened. They ordered an ultrasound of the IV site, which showed that I had formed a blood clot where the IV was.

A few hours went by, and once again my IV spot became red, hot and swollen, so they switched arms and put the IV in my right arm. Several hours passed, and it started happening again, so they ordered another ultrasound, which showed another blood clot. The doctor's plan turned from wanting to place a PICC line to wanting to place a Hickman port inside of my chest! This was way scarier than the PICC line to me, so I began to pray out, and I told God very specifically, "Lord, if this surgery is Your will, then please let it go okay, but if this surgery isn't Your will, please talk to the doctor and make him call it off." I told the doctor to schedule the Hickman line because I was placing my trust in God. The doctor also wanted the hematologist to come in to talk to me to see if we could find a safe blood thinner for me to take before the surgery because some blood thinners can be unsafe for Alpha-gal patients.

The next day the surgeon's assistant came into the room to go over the procedure, and right behind him came the surgeon. My husband had a few questions and also wanted to make sure the surgeon knew that I had mast cell activation syndrome and Alpha-gal syndrome. That way, they were aware of the risk of a reaction so they could be prepared. The surgeon then looked me in the eyes and said, "How much of this is even real?" In return my husband replied, "Excuse me?" The surgeon then proceeded to tell me that he felt this was just all in my head. My husband was quick to respond back that this was not in my head, that the doctor did not know what he was talking about and that these were actual documented medical conditions. The doctor then said, "I have never heard of these illnesses, and I don't believe those are even real conditions." He then looked at his assistant and said, "Let's go. They can find another surgeon to do her surgery. I am not wasting my time."

I was so hurt. How could he accuse me of making up not one but two medical diseases that were clearly documented? My doctor came back in, and at this point I was in tears and said, "You won't believe what that man said to me." My doctor said, "Don't even say it; there is no reason to repeat it. He already expressed his opinion to me. Don't worry about him." I later learned he wasn't the hospital's normal surgeon but rather an on-call surgeon from another hospital because of the holidays. It was Christmas/New Year's time, and the hematologist I had been seeing was gone.

So, my doctor decided to try things the oral route because we could no longer try an IV, due to the blood clots and the on-call surgeon refusing to put the port in, so he ordered pain medication and B1 thiamine. I knew that it wasn't a great plan, but what other options did I have? The nurse gave me the medications. I took them and fell asleep.

I woke up around midnight to a knot in my throat and my body broken out in a rash. I pressed my nurse's call button and asked for help. She came in and saw what was going on and went into a panic. She said, "Oh no, I can't handle this" and left the room to call the doctor. She returned with children's flavored Benadryl and told me to take it. I informed her that I have anaphylactic reactions to the dye alone in that medication but that I had an emergency pack of

71

compounded Benadryl in my purse that I could take if she would hand it to me. The hospital's policy was that I was not supposed to take my own medication from home but rather only what the hospital provided, but she handed it to me anyway.

It was not long after that when my doctor showed up. After talking to me for a minute he asked if he could call my husband. At this point it was past midnight. I said yes and he called and woke him up. He explained what was going on and felt that since everything we had tried at the hospital was going wrong, my husband should come pick me up and that being at home was my best option because I would be more comfortable.

The next morning my husband showed up to get me. At this point I was extremely sick and all of my nurses on staff that morning were surprised to see me go. Even though I hadn't known the medical staff for very long, being hospitalized for a period of time allowed me the chance to know them on a more personal level, and it was sad to say bye.

I remember the frosty breeze hitting my face for the first time in what had seemed like forever as they wheeled me out to the car, and I remember the brightness of the sun shining down on my face. I had wondered if I would make it out of the hospital alive to experience those feelings again.

As we were driving down the busy interstate, I stuck my hand out of the window. It was lightly snowing, and I could feel each little snowflake hit my hand, and it was so refreshing. I may have been dying and sick as could be, but even then, I was in awe of all the little beautiful things that God had made.

I have to say, even in the midst of the worst battles and hardships I have faced in my life, I can always find something beautiful in the storm. All I have to do is open my eyes and look around. I have come to realize we have two choices; we can choose to focus on the negative things in life, or we can choose to find the beauty in all situations. Even though it can be hard sometimes, I still choose to see the beauty in life.

Chapter 9

The Breakthrough

I had returned back home from the hospital for my own comfort as the doctor requested because there was nothing more the hospital could offer, and nothing was better. If anything, I was more hopeless than before. I just could not understand why none of the treatments were working. Why was my body rejecting everything? I was literately starving to death and in so much pain that life was becoming unbearable, and depression had really begun to set in. I had even begun to get angry toward God. Don't get me wrong; I love Him with all my heart, but I couldn't even begin to understand why I wasn't healed yet, and in that moment in time, He felt so far away that I just couldn't see how much He was truly working on my behalf.

I remember one morning I had found the strength to slide into my electric wheelchair (which I called "Frank") from the bed, and I wheeled myself to the back bedroom, where I just completely broke down. My mother-in-law had just walked in at the time, and I remember her just holding me as tears streamed down my face because I was not ready to die. I wanted to live no matter the fight. I was not ready to give up just yet.

I decided that I needed to refocus my thoughts on positive things, and I also decided to start confessing positive things in my life even when I could not see them. Some may find it silly, but from that moment on I confessed out loud every single day that I would walk again in the name of Jesus, and I would live and not die! I was not ignoring the symptoms I was going through, but I had to start confessing some type of goodness into my life. When I had doubts if I would ever walk again, I met it with a positive response that I would walk again!

During that time someone on a support group sent me a medical article on a natural mast cell stabilizer which they had been prescribed for mast cell activation syndrome. I had read about patients with MCAS being treated with medical cannabis, but I had not tried this medical treatment option because it was illegal in my state. I had come to the point though that if I didn't find a treatment or if God didn't come through with a miracle, I wasn't going to be here much longer, and the thought of not seeing my son grow up and not having the opportunity to grow older with my husband was more unbearable than the thought of being arrested for trying a scientifically proven mast cell stabilizer that could possibly save my life!

I decided I would show my husband all the medical research on the treatment option that was being offered to other mast cell patients in other states and countries and talk to him about giving this treatment a try because honestly what else did I have to lose? I was already losing my whole life in the most torturous way possible, and my weight had dropped to eighty-five pounds. I had experienced major muscle atrophy to the point where you could no longer feel any leg muscle; instead, you just felt bone and mushy skin all the way around. After reading through all the medical studies, we both agreed that we needed to give this option a try, but how would my doctors and family take the news of medical cannabis being a natural mast cell stabilizer? It was not offered legally in the state of Alabama, but how far would you go to save your life?

After talking it over, we decided that we would hold off on telling our family and friends about the medical treatment option that we were getting ready to try. We wanted to see first if it would even work or if my body would reject it, causing a reaction just as everything else we had previously tried, but finding organic medical cannabis in the state of Alabama proved very challenging, leaving us to have to venture out of state.

The time had finally come for me to try the organic medical cannabis, and I was so scared to try it as I did not know what to expect. I typically do not react well to breathing in vapors or fragrances of any kind, much less a thick cloud of smoke, but this was my chance to see if it would help or not, so I prayed and pushed past my fears, stepping out of my comfort zone, and tried it. It wasn't but moments until I could feel this cool, calming sensation pass over my entire body. At this moment I was in awe because I could literally feel my body calming down, and it was beyond amazing.

As we stepped up the amount of the medication to every hour, a large majority of the symptoms I was experiencing became more tolerable. Within moments the hives and skin flushing eased up. The horrible, sickening nausea eased up. The burning and inflammation in my GI tract began to ease up significantly. The uncontrollable tremors, muscle spasms and sweating eased up within moments, and the seizures I had been experiencing, which had totaled around forty at that moment in time, had come to a halt without having to take the seizure medication I was prescribed.

This was a major miracle for me. No, it wasn't a cure, and yes, I am still severely affected by mast cell activation syndrome, but this along with the compounded Benadryl had calmed my system enough for me to find a couple more safe foods and vitamins of a very specific brand that my body could keep down, thus helping me battle the extreme malnutrition stage I was facing.

After seeing that my body was tolerating this treatment option very well, we decided to open up to my doctors back in Alabama about how well the medical cannabis was working. We also decided to tell our family and friends, but to be able to explain how medical cannabis was helping to stabilize my mast cells, I had to first understand how our endocannabinoid system works.

I learned that the body's endocannabinoid system (ECS) involves a group of cell receptors and correlating molecules. Our ECS consists of two main cell receptors (CB1) and (CB2). To provide a better visual, we can imagine these cell receptors as locks on the exterior of cells and the chemical molecules called "agonists" as the key. Every time an agonist binds to a cell receptor, it sends information that results in a surge of chemical effects.

We can find CB1 receptors in our spinal cord and brain. CB2 receptors can be located in our immune cells of the peripheral nervous system.

Mast cells contain not one but both CB1 and CB2 receptors. Because of this, research shows us that cannabinoids (THC) will bind to these receptors suppressing mast cell degranulation.

Cannabinoids are broadly immunosuppressive, and anti-inflammatory properties have been reported for certain marijuana constituents and endogenously produced cannabinoids. The CB2 cannabinoid receptor is an established constituent of immune system cells, and we have recently established that the CB1 cannabinoid receptor is expressed in mast cells. (….). Taken together, these results reveal the complexity in signalling of natively co-expressed cannabinoid receptors and suggest that some anti-inflammatory effects of CB1 ligands may be attributable to sustained cAMP elevation that, in turn, causes suppression of mast cell degranulation (Small-Howard et al, 2005).

A leading mast cell activation syndrome expert, Dr. Lawrence Afrin, shares his experience with patients who use medical cannabis to help with their mast cell disease symptoms in his book *Never Bet Against Occam*:

> The mast cell surface features (inhibitory) cannabinoid receptors, making me wonder whether at least some of the chronically ill patients out there who claim that the only thing that makes them feel better is marijuana might be unrecognized MCAS patients in whom THC's binding with the

cannabinoid receptors on their dysfunctional mast cells leads to a quieting of the activity of those cells and thus a lessening of symptoms (Afrin, 2016. Pg. 436).

CBD alone without THC may be ineffective at treating dysfunctional mast cells because Tetrahydrocannabinol (THC) has a well-founded binding affinity for both CB1 and CB2 receptors. While Cannabidiol (CBD) may provide therapeutic benefits that are produced by indirect actions, CBD itself showed no distinct binding affinity.

"Cannabinomimetic Control of Mast Cell Mediator Release: New Perspective in Chronic Inflammation," published in *Journal of Neuroendocrinology,* provides detailed evidence backing up the fact that medical cannabis can suppress mast cell degranulation and help alleviate pain and inflammation in patients.

Now that I understood how medical cannabis worked as a mast cell stabilizer, I had to look into the ways that we could incorporate it into my medical routine. There were different options available, such as edibles, oils, ointments and smoking the actual flower itself, but in my case, my body has only tolerated smoking the organic medical cannabis flower, as the medical cannabis oil caused an allergic reaction when ingested because of the extraction process it takes to make the oil along with the MCT oil that is used to cut the oil.

We also tried the organic marijuana vaping oil, and at first it seemed to go okay, but after using it for a few days in a row, it built up and caused heart issues. And just like the edible oil, when the vape oil leaked from the tip of the cartridge onto my lips, it caused blisters and swelling in my lymph nodes. We also found out that I only tolerate the organic unbleached hemp rolling papers.

In the research study "Differential Roles of CB1 and CB2 Cannabinoid Receptors in Mast Cells," Maria-Teresa Samson (et al, 2003) stated:

> In the context of smoked marijuana, cannabinoids gain access to the systemic circulation within minutes of inhalation. However, airways and the gastrointestinal tract are immediate points of contact for cannabinoids constituents, and the resident mast cells in these areas will be impacted by marijuana smoke. Mast cells express CB2 cannabinoid receptors and a variety of responses to cannabinoid application have been described in these cells. In vitro, suppression of mast cell proinflammatory mediator release by both marijuana constituents and endocannabinoids has been described. The marijuana constituent tetrahydrocannabinol (THC)

is highly suppressive in vivo models of mast cell proinflammatory function.

When we came home from the hospital, we knew we had to step it up and keep trying new things, like stepping out to try the medical cannabis treatment option. We also felt that there just had to be something else out there that I hadn't tried to eat yet. So, my husband took off to the grocery store for what seemed like an endless, desperate search in trying to find something different that I could try. He came across a frozen package of wild caught Alaskan salmon and decided that since we had not tried any type of fish—and since it was alpha-gal free and raised in the wild—it might be a good place to start. We were both very excited but really nervous about this new potential protein source that he had found.

When trying something new, we have different steps that we go through.

Step one: a chew-and-spit test. A lot of times a simple chew and spit test can let me know if I am going to react to something, because sometimes I will develop symptoms (such as facial numbness or swelling of the lips, tongue or throat) within fifteen minutes of this test.

Step two; if I pass step one, then I move on to taking a small bite, swallowing and waiting a day. I do this because even though something may pass the chew-and-spit test, it doesn't mean it will pass actually swallowing and digesting it. This is typically the time I know if my body will accept or reject something.

Step three: if I pass the first two steps, we will slowly increase the intake amount of the new food/supplement/medication. Sometimes I may pass the first two tests with flying colors, but that still doesn't mean that my body will accept something. There are times where we have introduced new foods/medications/vitamins that appeared to do great at first, but after a few days of building up in my system on the said item, my body would start to reject it.

We also only introduced one thing at a time with several days in between, trying each new product. That way, if there was an issue, we knew exactly what was causing it.

My husband sautéed the wild caught Alaskan salmon he had found in nothing but my well water. We started with the spit test, and it did great! We were so surprised, so we moved on to the swallow test, and it stayed down and didn't cause my throat to swell! This was huge to us. A little time went by of my body holding down the salmon. This showed us that there were possibly still some things out there that my body would tolerate. So, he went back to the store and made a list of everything organic that I had not tried. While he was there, he decided to pick up a pack of GreenWise Organic

Chicken, as it was a different brand than the chicken I had tried from a different store and reacted to.

We were a little nervous about this because the same brand also has an all-natural chicken that my body has reacted to on numerous occasions, even when boiled in my safe water with nothing added. But this time we were holding onto hope that maybe something would be different, and it was! Like the salmon, the organic chicken stayed down and didn't cause any throat or facial swelling! This was a win for me. I knew that the two new meats had to help the malnutrition.

We decided, since I had responded well to the GreenWise Organic Chicken, to give some of the other organic GreenWise products a try. He went back to the store and picked up GreenWise Organic Oats, black beans, green beans, and corn. We started with the oats cooked in my well water with nothing else added, and to our surprise, it went well. This was good news because I had already tried another brand of oatmeal, which made me sick. Here I was with two new meats and an oatmeal that were doing well.

Next, we were very eager to try the green beans, as we knew I needed something green in my diet, but almost immediately following the spit test my bubble came to a shattering pop as my throat began to swell, I became very numb in the face and my body started vomiting and dry-heaving even though I hadn't even swallowed anything.

At this point, although I had been able to tolerate the other things, emotionally I was back at step one, heartbroken and still sick. But after a few days of allowing my system to recover and just eating the chicken, salmon and oatmeal and using the cannabis around the clock every hour, I regained the strength to try something new again.

This time, I tried the corn just because I liked corn more than black beans, but it basically ended in the same dramatic scenario as it had with the green beans. After this I became hesitant because it was very clear that even though I was tolerating the salmon, chicken and oats, my reactions were still very much real and just as scary as they ever were.

It's a feeling that's so hard to describe, not knowing if you're going to be able to find anything to eat at all and knowing that the next bite of something new could be a violent or deadly reaction, but at the same time you know if you don't try new things the path that you're currently on would lead to an agonizing death as well. So, through a lot of prayer and support from my husband, I decided about a week later to give the black beans a shot, and can I say hallelujah! After two miserable fails with the other vegetables, the black beans showed no signs of any reaction (and I had already tried another brand of organic black beans that previous year which had caused a reaction).

Over the course of the next couple of months, we continued down the same path, trying one-ingredient organic items one by one, and had more failures than successes. For example, Publix carried organic frozen blueberries, raspberries, strawberries and mixed berries, all of which caused violent reactions except for the blueberries, which I can eat all day long. There were a few successes that were oh so important.

So, after learning all of this and proceeding with the new medical treatment, a couple more months passed, and I had slowly been able to add in a few safe foods and supplements to my diet, but just to give you a clear picture, my diet is very limited to these exact brands, as other brands we have tried (even of the same products) have caused anaphylactic reactions:

- GreenWise Organic Chicken (the all-natural chicken still caused a reaction, and when we looked into why this might have happened, we discovered that one is chilled in an antibacterial water solution versus the other is immediately flash-frozen)
- GreenWise Organic Black Beans
- GreenWise Organic Oats
- GreenWise Organic Frozen Spinach

- GreenWise Organic Frozen Blueberries
- GreenWise Organic Unrefined Coconut Oil
- GreenWise Organic Maple Syrup (in the glass bottle)
- Frozen wild caught Alaskan salmon
- GreenWise Organic Ketchup

The GreenWise Organic Ketchup is the most puzzling thing I can eat due to it being the only multiple-ingredient item on my list. It contains Organic** tomatoes, sugar, vinegar, salt and spices, all of which I react to when used separately even store-bought tomatoes would cause a reaction although I do tolerate a specific band of canned diced tomatoes. For example, we haven't been able to find any salt that doesn't make me sick besides what's in this ketchup, and the same goes for the rest of these ingredients.

So, basically, it's blueberry oatmeal for breakfast, chicken or salmon served with black beans and spinach as sides for lunch and dinner every day. Now, I know that seems like something I would get tired of, but the truth is that it is way better than the flour and water noodles and diced tomatoes that I had lived off of for the previous year any day, and I am still trying to find new foods to add. It's a long, slow process, but I am hoping to one day have a little larger variety of foods, and if for some reason I don't, well, God is good all the time, and I am beyond grateful for my oatmeal, blueberries, spinach, beans, chicken and well water.

As far as supplements, just like with food I am very limited to certain products of certain brands. But even then we are running into the problem with manufacturers changing the ingredients, resulting in my body tolerating one supplement one minute but not the next. We are still fighting to get a steady source of vitamins and supplements that are vital for my health, such as:

- Vitamin A
- Vitamin C
- Vitamin B Complex
- Vitamin E
- Vitamin D
- Magnesium
- Calcium
- Zinc
- Potassium
- Iodine
- Iron

If you are wondering why I am being so specific here, it is because these specific details may help save someone who is also battling with mast cell activation syndrome and hasn't been able to find a safe food that they can tolerate. I truly believe one of the most important keys to surviving this disease is making sure that we keep our nutrition under control, and in my case, that wasn't the easiest of tasks.

Thanks to the new medical treatment plan calming my body down enough to tolerate the few safe foods I had found, I slowly started gaining a little weight back, going from 85 lbs to 101 lbs. We decided to open up to my doctors in Alabama and family.

We started with my doctors. I was extremely nervous about even mentioning it to them because I did not know how they would respond, but after opening up to my doctors, they were very receptive and told me they could see a major difference and that they recommended I keep taking the medical cannabis as I had been because the improvement was that drastic.

After seeing how positive my medical professionals handled the news, we decided to call my immediate family to our house to tell them all about the medical treatments I was receiving, and at this point I was even more nervous than I had been when it was time to tell the doctors. I guess I was scared that they would judge my choice of medical treatment instead of accepting it. So, I made sure I had every medical study I could find on medical cannabis and mast cell activation syndrome printed off and lying on the table for them to read, along with the mast cell specialist book page marked to the information on the subject just so they could not refute anything I was saying, but to my surprise they were extremely accepting and said that they had noticed a major difference and were so happy that I found a medical treatment that was saving my life because that was what mattered—being here with the people I loved and making new memories.

Chapter 10

Living in an Illegal State

We finally had begun to see a light at the end of a very long dark tunnel, and we were so grateful because our prayers were being met. God had opened up so many doors to get me to a point where I was able to slowly heal from all the damage that had occurred from the severe malnutrition and dehydrated state I had been in because of the mast cell activation syndrome, but the fears of my life-saving medication being illegal in my state were very real and scary even though my medical illness was covered under a medical defense law called "Leni's Law," allowing the use of medical cannabis oil with low THC. However, that oil did not help me because, like I mentioned before, I am allergic to the oil and can only tolerate the organic medical marijuana flower itself.

This law is amazing for giving some patients a defense in court regarding certain medical conditions, but mast cell activation syndrome isn't so simple, as some patients do not tolerate the medical cannabis oils but can tolerate smoking the organic medical cannabis flower itself and need a stronger amount of THC then this defense law allows.

So, even though mast cell activation syndrome is protected under a defense law to a certain percentage, it is not enough, as it doesn't cover the medical treatment options of medical cannabis that is required to control mast cell activation syndrome, leaving patients very vulnerable to not only the fear and consequences of facing jail time but also the great risk of anaphylaxis (which could lead to death) from the jail's environment. Not to mention the jail would not have a safe food or water supply for them to survive on. All of this could result just because patients needed their life-saving medication. Additionally, mast cell activation syndrome patients cannot just get medical cannabis off of the streets because of the risk of contamination.

Cannabis off of any street corner can be laced with anything, and it can also be grown with pesticides and fertilizers that can cause anaphylactic reactions in mast cell patients, so in order for mast cell patients to have proper medical cannabis to treat their condition, it needs to be grown organically and distributed in a sterile environment.

Because of this, mast cell activation syndrome patients, along with many others, have to travel out of state for medical treatment, myself included. This is no easy feat as it can uproot your loved one's lives as well as your own, and it is very costly. Not only do you have to have the money to cover the cost of treatment, as insurance doesn't cover it, but also the cost of living while you are out of state. This also isn't easy for a mast cell patient on disability who has to have specific foods like me that may not be offered in the new state that you are staying in while receiving treatment. There are a lot of hoops to jump through to get there, such as filling up gallons of your safe water and a week's worth of your safe foods to take with you because none of the stores in the other states offer those things, leaving your family to make multiple trips between states because your water and food only last a week—maybe two at the max. Then there is always the major risk of loved ones being pulled over while driving across the country to get your medicine, putting their own lives on the line because they believe you are worth saving. There are so many other life-altering hoops to jump through that I could mention here, but the point is if it means saving your life, well, you are worth saving no matter the cost because there is not another person like you.

I was so excited to learn that there was a push to legalize medical cannabis in my home state. I even took the time to reach out with my story to the very ones trying to pass the bill along with the state representatives, hoping that they would add in my situation so it would be covered under the new bill, but I was very saddened when I realized after it

93

passed the bill only applied to medical cannabis oils. Like I mentioned before, ingesting the medical cannabis oils may trigger anaphylactic reactions in mast cell patients, but smoking the organic medical cannabis flower itself has shown to be better tolerated, thus lessening symptoms and bringing the condition under better control. In my case, the medical cannabis oils caused anaphylactic symptoms when I ingested them or used the vape oils, along with causing blisters to form on my lips and in my mouth. However, my body does tolerate smoking the organic medical cannabis flower itself, giving me the chance to get the MCAS under control enough to survive this horrible illness.

I remember sitting there in shock the morning I found out that the bill had passed. How could the representatives and the governor possibly see the medical benefits of a medication that is scientifically proven to help control a condition that can be very life-threatening but tell you that you cannot receive this proven life-saving treatment legally because it is not in a processed oil form? That sounds silly, doesn't it? And it is a prime example of discrimination against someone's disability and his or her civil rights. I mean, what does it matter if it is in oil form or flower form if it is saving a young mother from an early grave or a small child from having seizures every day? It shouldn't matter and should be available to all the people who need it to survive in the form of treatment their individual bodies tolerate, whether that be medical cannabis oil or the medical flower itself.

Picture this: a lady is driving home after picking up her medical cannabis oil for depression and she is pulled over. The cop finds the medical cannabis oil; he proceeds to ask for her medical marijuana card and then lets her go because she has proof that she is medically supposed to have this medication and therefore it is perfectly legal.

Now imagine a young mother driving home after picking up her proven life-saving organic medical marijuana flower because she cannot tolerate the medical marijuana oil itself due to the extraction process and her disability, and all of a sudden she is pulled over, except this time the cop isn't so nice. Because the marijuana flower itself is not covered under the new bill, this stop results in this young mother being arrested, charged with a felony and treated like a criminal!

How does this even remotely begin to sound fair? It's not fair. How can you say to one person, "You can have your medical marijuana oil and be safe without the risk of criminal charges" but tell the other person who has to have the unprocessed organic medical marijuana flower to actually survive a rare disease that they can't? How can you not offer the same legal protection to both patients?

Honestly, this was exactly what the state was doing to me. They were telling patients with depression that they could legally have the marijuana oils but were telling me that I could not have this scientifically proven mast cell stabilizer in the form that my body accepted which brought me up off of my deathbed. This not only sounds like discrimination of my disability, but it also goes against my civil rights!

I have the right to equal protection just as much as other patients!

I do not keep up with politics, as I have too much going on, but I did see the claim in an article regarding the medical cannabis debate that there was no such thing as medical cannabis and patients could find it on the streets in my state, thus cancelling the need to legalize it for medical use. I want to clarify that this statement is just not true. As mentioned before, mast cell patients have to be extremely careful of contamination as well as what the plant was grown in, because if this medical plant was not grown in the proper sterile environment, it could cause allergic-type reactions in MCAS patients, and because there are many different strains of medical cannabis, MCAS patients must be careful to obtain the right one. Some strains help mast cell patients greatly while others may not, which is why mast cell patients truly need a place to get their organically grown medical cannabis in the form that their body tolerates, whether it be the flower or the oil, in a safe environment where they can get a steady flow of the medical cannabis strain they need, even if that means they have to grow it themselves.

I have also seen where several DAs sent their own letters to lawmakers, opposing medical marijuana and stating, "Marijuana is a wolf in sheep's clothing." I found that kind of ironic because the same thing could be said about some DAs as well. Some of these individuals think that marijuana is a gateway drug and that it shouldn't be legal. I think that they are forgetting that marijuana can be found on any street corner if someone truly wants it.

At the end of the day, the only ones who are being hurt by this are the sick and the helpless. Since anyone can get cannabis off any street corner, then what would it hurt to legalize the medical marijuana flower to help the sick get the proper organically grown strain that their bodies may need? And, yes, there is such a thing as medical-grade cannabis, as I previously stated.

It still surprises me that there's so much pushback against this life-saving medical herb that is our God-given right to try and that patients are being arrested for it and booked with harsher bail amounts than dangerous criminals!

Alabama has a growing problem with methamphetamines that is ruining families and lives every single day, but we are remaining silent to that fact, and their meth addiction did not start from needing the medical marijuana flower to survive. It started with them making a choice to administer addicting toxic poisons into their bodies, not one of God's medicinal herbs—do not get that confused!

If these DAs truly want to make a difference, then they should stop pressing criminal charges against the sick and helpless that need the medical marijuana flower and start throwing the hammer down on what is really destroying lives—methamphetamines, crack cocaine, opium prescription medicine abuse, and even alcohol! Put your efforts into cleaning the methamphetamines, crack cocaine and pharmaceutical pills up off of our streets! That's where you will make the greatest impact, and you should have more room in the jails and prisons to house the methamphetamine and crack cocaine dealers along with more room in rehabs for those who are addicted to these terrible drugs.

The reality of the situation likely comes down to money. If the system makes more money off of marijuana offenses than it does off of methamphetamines or crack cocaine, then why would they want to make it medically legal? How would the court system make more money? Marijuana users are typically good people with jobs that will pay all the fees that the court orders them to pay, versus those on illicit drugs rarely have a sense of responsibility or morals and will spend all their money on drugs and will choose to go on the run, hiding from the law instead of paying the fines that the court has ordered them to pay! This isn't even mentioning those who might personally profit from the medical cannabis flower not being legalized.

Heck, to take it a step further, if the DAs truly wanted to make our streets safer then they would stop letting violent pedophiles back out on the streets and start giving them harsher sentences! While we're at it, why stop there?

Every year an estimated 300,000 children are taken worldwide and are sold by human traffickers for purposes such as prostitution, marriage, forced labor, and, in some cases, adoption and organ removal, while the media and government seem to remain silent.

According to the International Labour Organization (ILO), an estimated 1.2 million children are trafficked each year. While human trafficking potentially earns global profits of an estimated $150 billion per year for human traffickers, an estimated $99 billion of that profit is brought in by commercial sexual exploitation!

Ready for the mind-blower? In the United States, reports show that a large portion of child sex trafficking victims were once in the foster care system! The very system that was created to protect them, but yet medical marijuana in flower form is what everyone has a problem with?

I do, however, have faith that God can and will move hearts in the great state of Alabama, and I am praying that the state representatives and the governor will show mercy upon the patients like me who truly need this life-saving medical treatment option. I can imagine the day where I can be home and feel safe again, not having to worry about traveling to a different state to receive treatment options or feel like I will be judged by others or risk going to jail all because of an illness I never asked for in the first place that all stems from a simple tick bite.

For the past two years we have reached out multiple times to the representatives who were trying to get a medical marijuana bill passed in Alabama as well as every other representative in the state that I could find an email for, only to be ignored. Well, CAN YOU HEAR ME NOW? I may not be able to walk into one of your meetings to make my voice heard because of my disability, but I can promise you that I am only going to get LOUDER until I can finally be safely at home again with my family without worrying if I'm going to be arrested or worse.

Writing this book alone for you to read puts a huge target on my back and creates a very dangerous situation for me, so please know I do not take stepping out with my story lightly. The fact is, there are people who would rather I die than legalize medical marijuana in smokeable form in

Alabama, and they proved that by choosing to ignore me, acting as if my life didn't matter to them.

Honestly though, I am more afraid of remaining silent, because by remaining silent I'm making myself just as bad as they are. Not only would remaining silent hurt myself and my family, but it would also hurt the countless others who cannot speak up for themselves at the moment.

The new bill that the governor just signed is called the "Compassion Act," which is said to provide safe usage and accesses to medical marijuana oil for qualifying patients, but where is the compassion for my situation? Where is the compassion for others who are like me? Because I can promise you I am not the only one.

Do we not also deserve the right to safely use and access medical marijuana in the form our bodies tolerate?

Do our lives not matter?

I pray every day that my life could just go back to normal or what used to be normal. I would love it, and I'm sure that a lot of other patients who need this medication to function feel the same way. Heck, I would love it if my body could tolerate the medical cannabis oil, but unfortunately it doesn't.

We do not want to have to use this medication. We did not choose these illnesses, but we will fight to choose to live, and we would love if you would stand with us to fight to make this life-saving medication legal in all its forms to all who truly need it. Would you please stand with us?

Chapter 11

That Bubble Life!

The past few years have been crazy. I feel like I have been through so much that most people could never even comprehend without having to go through it themselves. Through all of this I feel like I have learned so much about life and myself. I choose to believe that all of this heartache has made me a better person, a more compassionate person. Most of all I have learned to trust in God's timing and not my own.

It has been three years now since I was crying out from my deathbed for the Lord to save me, and oh, how He has. It may not be a picture-perfect completely gone miraculous healing, but by His mercies I get to wake up each day with my amazingly beautiful family.

I have to stick to a very strict schedule and live life as if I am quarantined inside of a bubble. Honestly, I guess I am quarantined away from the world, and even though I have had to give up so much, such as the simple freedom of going on shopping trips and even just hanging out with friends, in the end I am completely okay with that because I am here, alive and not in the grave.

My daily routine consists of eating the same three meals a day. I start with a hot, yummy bowl of organic oats with blueberries followed by organic chicken, spinach and black beans for lunch and dinner. I know it may seem like it would get tiring to eat the same three meals a day, but two years ago I was surviving only on diced tomatoes and flour noodles, which almost killed me, so being able to eat these three hot real meals a day is beyond a miracle. It is an answered prayer that I am thankful for every time I get to sit down at the dinner table with my family.

I know what it feels like to literately starve to death, so you will never hear me complain about my safe foods. Every time I sit down to take a bite, a refreshing feeling of happiness overtakes my soul, and I am beyond grateful. It even still brings tears to my eyes. Before I was forcing myself to eat the bitter diced tomatoes and flour noodles, but now, I absolutely look forward to sitting down to eat my meal, and I savor every single bite as if it's the first. There is just a complete sense of thankfulness that completely overtakes me, and I don't think one can comprehend that until the basic necessities in life, such as eating a simple meal, drinking a glass of water or simply just walking outdoors to sit in the sunshine, is taken away.

When it comes to our household routine, the type of dish soap we use and the material that the dishes are made of are very important. We have found that even if my safe food is cooked in (or with anything) other than stainless steel or glass, it can cause an allergic response, and so far the only dish soap we have found that my body tolerates is Seventh Generation Free & Clear, but even then my dishes have to be washed extremely well and overly rinsed because any residue left behind has also shown to trigger an extremely severe allergic response in my body that lasts for several days.

Next is the laundry. This was actually a hard one to overcome as I am beyond crazy allergic to basically any chemical perfumed scents including laundry soaps, fabric softener, shampoos, and even some people's deodorants. But after searching, we finally found one laundry soap that my clothes can be washed in that doesn't cause me issues to wear—All Free Clear.

Before I became sick, I can remember dousing myself in perfume or body spray anytime I was going somewhere. I loved to smell amazing, but I never once thought about the health effects that my perfume or fabric softeners could cause someone else to go through. If I would have known the things that I now know, I would have done things completely differently not only for someone else's health but also for my own, as many perfumes, lotions and laundry soaps on the market are full of toxic chemicals that are proven to harm our bodies, and I was completely blinded to that at the time.

Because the mast cell activation syndrome still has my diet very limited and therefore restricts the nutrition that I need, I have to supplement that with vitamins. I previously mentioned the vitamins I was advised to take, they totaled up to fourteen different vitamin pills a day, which is a lot harder than you might think. I actually have to have someone in the room when I take pills or eat because I still struggle to swallow, but it is a lot better than having an artificial tube placed in my chest with the risk of reacting to the TPN ingredients.

My body must have THC around the clock to function. If not, my mast cells become more irritated and activated, increasing symptoms, leading to a downward spiral in my health and causing me to lose the battle I am fighting so hard each day to win.

With the combination of THC (from the medical cannabis flower) around the clock, compounded Benadryl when needed and the daily intake of vitamins that I can tolerate, I have found a routine that has helped me start to better control the mast cell activation syndrome. Even though I am still extremely sensitive, at least I can finally catch a breath of fresh air.

I have to social distance myself from others because of the different chemical fragrances that most people have on, which often causes my throat to swell along with other symptoms. Heck, I've even had reactions to groceries that my husband brought home because the lady who bagged them had scented lotion on her hands, leaving behind scented residue on all our groceries. Or the fact that someone's cigarette smoke tends to travel in the air, causing once again another reaction. And there are many more examples I could give.

Losing the ability to go out and do something with friends has been hard at times, even with my husband and son by my side, because it can get lonely, but I am so content because I am here breathing—something that I wouldn't have dreamed I would be doing if you had told me I'd be here three years ago.

I have made so many new friends from all across the world who are fighting a similar battle as me, if not the same. Countless people have reached out to me after hearing my story, which has opened doors to be able to share God's love in ways I didn't even think were possible as well as offering the knowledge of the things that I have learned so far and having the opportunity to hear things that they have learned as well. That being said, I have also lost many new friends to this disease, which is beyond hard in itself. I find myself just breaking down into tears if I think about it too hard, but at least I was able to meet them and share His love and kindness with them while I had the chance.

To be honest, I'm not sure why I am still here winning an uphill battle I face every single day and some of my friends are gone, but I do know that it makes me want to push to create a change, to be a voice in this world to make us heard, if not only for them and myself but also for the countless others who are suffering due to lack of knowledge.

While I was on my deathbed, there was another person around my age in a hospital across the country who was also suffering from mast cell activation syndrome and tick-borne disease, fighting the same battle as me, at the same time as me. If I were to put our stories side by side, they would be almost identical, but she went on to be with Jesus.

I hold this person very close to my heart because it reminds me that every single second of life is a blessing and a chance to show kindness in this world and that this life is so fragile. I choose to remember her and others like her so they are not forgotten. Their stories encourage me to take better actions to try to help educate the medical community and patients about the dangers of tick-borne diseases and mast cell activation syndrome.

You may be shocked to know, but in the great state of Alabama, 90% of the medical community that I had spoken with, including specialists, family practitioners and nurses, had not even heard of mast cell activation syndrome before, and a large majority were very uneducated on tick-borne diseases and how to diagnose and provide proper treatment.

It's a sad fact, but many patients affected by tick-borne diseases or mast cell activation syndrome are often labeled as crazy, being told it's "all in your head" and "antidepressants should help," all because their doctors are uneducated on the matter. Many patients have even been admitted to psych wards against their will, and if you think this couldn't possibly happen to you, think again.

When this all started, I heard so many crazy things like "it's anxiety," so I asked, "Does anxiety make your face and throat swell?"

The allergist said, "Well, no, it wouldn't. Honestly I can't give you an answer because it's over my head."

And then we could even go back to the surgeon who refused to do my surgery because my conditions were "made up" in my head because he had never heard of them.

I've been told often that I am too pretty to be sick or that I don't look sick because I'm pretty. This is mind-blowing to me because I didn't know that being pretty makes you invincible to illnesses. Sounds like a very silly

109

statement, doesn't it? And I have been asked if I was anorexic! Which my answer is "Absolutely not. I love food and I would never intentionally make myself sick!" If I could I would be eating a medium-rare steak, baked potatoes, salad and a big fat piece of chocolate cake. Don't tell me I don't like to eat.

So, when I talk about being a voice this is the exact reason why. Too many patients are being tossed aside because of the medical community not providing enough education on the subject, thus leading patients to experience hardships, harassment, and increased sickness due to lack of treatment. I now suffer from PTSD because of everything I went through at the hands of unknowledgeable doctors, and due to the stress of watching me slowly die, my husband also shows signs of PTSD when in certain situations.

Surprisingly, I spoke with one doctor who specialized in sports injuries and, to my surprise, he told me that he had to do a thirty-minute study on mast cell activation syndrome while in school. He admitted he didn't know that much about it, but at least this condition is finally starting to be taught in school.

If you're like me, when this all first started, you were probably clueless regarding what to look for in a healthcare provider. I would suggest looking for someone who is knowledgeable in both functional and naturopathic medicine.

Keep in mind that the doctor works for you, not the other way around. It is always good to take someone with you to help serve as your advocate. You should never feel ignored, bullied or harassed by your doctor or their staff members. If you have found yourself in this position, then it is time to find a new healthcare provider.

When looking for a new medical professional, it is important to find someone who truly cares for their patients, taking the time to actually sit down with them, showing compassion and truly listening to what's going on instead of making them feel like it's "anxiety, or it's all in your head."

You need someone who will come in to spend an hour with you if needed, not someone who walks in for fifteen minutes, only to push pills at you. Your doctor should be someone who looks for the root cause of the problems; you do not want a doctor who only tries to cover the problems up with pills like a Band-Aid. Most of the time some of the medications they prescribe can cause a whole list of side effects of their own. A good doctor can be hard to find, but they are out there, so don't give up.

We need the medical community to become more aware and educated on mast cell activation syndrome and tick-borne diseases not only to help keep patients from suffering but also because there are not very many doctors who specialize in this field, leaving patients with only a handful of specialists to choose from, some of whom have a history of picking and choosing their patients based on the severity of their illnesses, accepting the easier cases and turning the most severe away, all the while still charging top dollar. This may not be true for all specialists, but nevertheless it is still happening.

So, please remember there are doctors and nonprofits who are there to make money, and then there are doctors and nonprofits who are there to truly help. You have to have discernment between the two.

Every day, I wake up in awe that I am alive. I may not be able to live a normal life and I may have to stay in my bubble on a very strict schedule, but oh, how there is always beauty in the storm. You just have to be willing to see it.

Since developing this illness, I feel like my eyes have been opened to a whole new world around me, and honestly it can be a scary sight. I was poisoning my body daily from consuming the toxins that are found in our food and water supplies. Sometimes I wonder if I would have remained blinded to this fact had it not been for this illness.

My husband jokes around and calls me his little canary, as they used canaries as warning signs in the coal mines to detect the presence of any toxic gas, which would let people know to leave before it could hurt them. He says that my body reacting to the toxins in our food and water supplies and the environment has opened his eyes to become more aware of what he was exposing not only himself to but our son as well.

In truth, after learning and going through everything that I have, I feel like a canary, even to the point of almost losing my life. My prayer is that this experience may open the eyes of others to see the dangerous territories that we are truly living in. Our food and water supplies as well as our hygiene products and our environment are being poisoned right in front of our eyes daily, and we are walking around blind to this fact. All the while childhood cancer, autism rates and reproductive issues are skyrocketing, but no one is questioning why.

I recently read an article called "Plummeting Sperm Counts, Shrinking Penises. Toxic Chemicals Threaten Humanity" by Erin Brockovich, where she went into a discussion about a book that was written by an environmental and reproductive epidemiologist named Shanna Swan. In this book called *Countdown*, Swan talks about the chemicals found in our cleaning and hygiene products as well as in our food and water supplies and how these chemicals are affecting our fertility and sperm count.

According to Erin Brockovich's article, Swan's book discusses her findings, and it was very alarming! It states that since 1973, men's sperm counts have decreased by up to 60%! Her research showed that unless we do something to take action now, by 2045, sperm counts could decrease to ZERO percent!

This should be very alarming to you, especially if you're looking forward to having grandchildren and great grandchildren one day, as I hope to. Now is the time to correct our mistakes to leave behind a better world for our future generations. We need to step back to take a look at the bigger picture and ask ourselves, "What kind of world are we creating to leave behind for them?"

Chapter 12

Nutrition! Nutrition! Nutrition!

Now, I know that we have talked a little about vitamins and minerals in the previous chapters, but I would like to take a moment to stress the importance of proper nutrition and hydration and how nutrients affect our bodies. To start with, what are nutrients? Nutrients are vitamins, minerals, water, fats, proteins and carbohydrates that provide our bodies with the nourishment that we need to function.

We get nutrients from the foods and liquids that we put into our bodies; the sun also provides us with vitamin D. So, if you have ever heard the saying "You are what you eat," this statement is beyond true. Everything that you put into your body is either helping to fight disease or it is helping to cause it.

While going through some medical research articles, I read that 92% of Americans suffer from at least one nutritional deficiency, and when it comes to the mast cell activation syndrome and Alpha-gal syndrome communities, multiple nutritional deficiencies are all too common. This is due to the restricted diets that patients may face, creating an extremely dangerous situation that can turn life-threatening in the blink of an eye.

Are nutritional deficiencies really that bad? The answer is YES! Nutritional deficiencies can cause problems that can range from something small such as brittle nails, dry skin and hair loss all the way to neuropathy, paralysis, blindness and even death.

To better help give you an example of how being undernourished and dehydrated can affect your body, I will share a few issues I've been through with malnutrition:

- Because I was not getting any Iodine in my diet this caused Iodine deficiency which possibly caused my thyroid to stop working properly creating a condition called hypothyroidism.

- Due to a Thiamine deficiency, I was experiencing extremely severe burning peripheral neuropathy, loss of feeling, paralysis of parts of my lower extremities. The Neuropathy even made its way into the palms of my hands.

- I was experiencing painful muscle cramps in my hands, legs and feet, which turned out to be caused by a potassium deficiency.

- I experienced sores on the corner of my mouth and a raw swollen tongue that wouldn't heal, hair loss, brittle nails, anxiety, depression and brain fog—all of which can be caused by an iron deficiency as well as a wide range of vitamin deficiencies (B1, B2, B6, B3, B7, B12)

- Iron deficiency symptoms also include shortness of breath, unusual craving for things such as ice, weakness and fatigue, headaches, dizziness, fast heartbeat, cold hands and feet, brittle nails and pale skin.
- Vitamin D deficiency can cause bone and joint pains, muscle pains and cramps, fatigue, mood changes, excessive sweating, digestive problems, immune impairments, low bone density and hair loss.

During the worst moments in my battle with malnutrition, my vision started to correct itself. I've always had to have a pair of glasses to see, but the sicker I became the better my vision got. Then I started having double vision, and at one point in time I went completely blind to details for ten minutes or so with glasses on. All I could see was a blurred green and blue blob of what should have been green trees and a beautiful blue sky.

I asked my eye specialist if they had heard of this before, and their theory was that my eyes were shrinking from the malnutrition and dehydration, causing my vision to become better, and that it was not a good thing. We also learned that a thiamine deficiency can cause severe vision loss.

As we slowly learned to get my nutrition under control, my vision started to get blurry again, and I now must wear glasses again to see. A multitude of the other symptoms I was experiencing due to malnutrition and dehydration started to correct itself.

Finding vitamins and supplements that my body would tolerate was one of the most crucial steps in this battle I faced. It was not a simple task, as we had to go through multiple reactions and supplements before we found the ones that I could take. It was all worth it though, pushing through and not giving up on finding oral supplements, because the option of a TPN was not looking so great for me as my body already didn't tolerate some of the ingredients in the TPN. So, pushing ingredients that I have already reacted to through my veins did not make much sense to me personally.

This little bit of information on nutrition is not even the tip of the iceberg. I could write a whole book on the subject. I encourage you to do some research yourself, as learning about proper nutrition will be one of the best decisions that you can make in your life, as lack of knowledge can literally be lack of life!

Chapter 13

The Priest, the Levite or the Good Samaritan?

Before, I had asked God how I was supposed to be normal like other Christians if I could not even simply step inside of a church building without experiencing an anaphylactic reaction because of the cleaning chemicals and fog machines used inside of the church. Over the past couple of years I have since learned that that's not what it is about at all.

You see, it's not about the church building, as the building itself will rot away someday. It's not about the next big revival meeting, as all you have to do to be revived is seek Him—and to be honest, I've felt God's presence just as strong, if not even stronger, while on my hands and knees seeking Him in my bathroom floor just as much as I have at a revival meeting. God will meet you where you are at. It's so important to remember that. It's not about being perfect. It's not about standing in the spotlight, preaching behind a podium. And for me personally, I would rather be in the background instead of standing in the spotlight any day.

It's simply just about being in a relationship with your Abba Father. Then, next thing you know, your heart is filled with His love and His kindness, which then just radiates into the world. And for it to do that, you don't have to preach down anyone's throat. You don't have to be inside of a church building every Wednesday and Sunday. Heck, you don't have to be perfect, because we all make mistakes and fall short of His glory every day (I know that I do, anyway). But the beautiful thing is that even with all my flaws, Jesus still thinks that I am golden, and He feels the same way about you.

Don't get me wrong; I'm not saying that attending regular church service isn't good, because it is wonderful. If you have a church family that is supportive and in a healthy relationship with Christ, then you have something precious and probably the most cherished treasure there is. All I am saying is don't think or teach that it is a necessary step to enter the kingdom of heaven. Christ will meet you wherever you are, as if you were the one on the cross right beside Him.

All we really have to do to shine His light in others' lives is care, take time to put a smile on our faces and listen to them. Be there for others because showing the love of Christ in all situations is the only thing that truly matters, and honestly that's easier said than done, believe me.

Truthfully, I have been through some tough things in my life, starting with my biological egg donor abandoning me not long after she had me, experiencing physical abuse at a young age, then going through multiple different stepmother figures who were not the nicest women especially when my dad wasn't around, one of whom fed me hard street drugs daily starting when I was just thirteen years old, which eventually led me to overdosing at the age of 13. That's when I had my first unexplainable, undeniable supernatural encounter with God as He reached out His piercing bright hand to pull me out of a place of total utter darkness. I'm not sure where I was exactly, but all I know is that the darkness was so dark that when I held my hand up to the tip of my nose, I literally could not see it.

I guess you could say I truly lived the life of Cinderella. I finally moved out on my own with my boyfriend (who is now my husband of sixteen wonderful years) when I wasn't even fifteen yet just to get away from her toxic environment, and that really doesn't even began to cover a fraction of the things I have been through in my short little life along with developing a crazy illness after a tick bite that has taken most of my life away, including suffering through the heartbreaking loss of not one but multiple miscarriages because of it.

The crazy things I have been through in my life would completely astonish you, but those stories would fill an entire book on their own. The point is that I have never had an easy life, but I was also never promised one. I chose to let every single thing I have been through make me a better person instead of carrying the weight, pain and bitterness inside.

I chose to be a good mom. I chose to turn away from drugs as soon as I left home as a young teen and turn away anyone who did them. I chose to remove toxic friends and family from my life, and I choose every day to wake up and put a smile on my beautiful little face because I know no matter what comes my way, I got this. I will choose to fight instead of giving up, and most of all I choose to focus on the happy things in life and making new memories even if I am trapped inside of a bubble.

I choose to have the mindset of a victor instead of a victim, and I choose to focus on the joyful things in life. Just because my world has been turned upside down doesn't mean my smile should be. We just had to learn to adjust to our circumstances and find the beauty and adventure in where we are now.

Things happen in life, and sometimes those things are not fair, but how we choose to respond to those things will make a drastic difference in the outcome of the battles we may face. We can choose to rise above the obstacles and keep fighting, or we can choose to surrender and give up. I had to personally learn to press through the physical pain, lay down the fears of the unknown and press toward hope that God wasn't finished with me yet if I wanted to survive.

One thing's for sure: just like when Daniel was thrown into a den with hungry lions or when Jonah was swallowed up in the belly of a fish or when Shadrach, Meshach and Abednego were thrown into the fire—and let's not forget about when the Apostle John was thrown into boiling oil—those terrible and frightening situations arose and may have not been fair, but in the midst of it all God was still there, working miracles.

God was with me too while I had been desperately searching for a proper specialist. Some of my family and friends started a fundraiser to help with travel, testing and treatment costs because my insurance would cover nothing done out of state. During this time complete strangers from all over the world took the time out of their busy lives to contact me just to talk or offer prayer and encouragement, while others reached out to let me know that I was not alone. I was completely blown away at the support and kindness that came flooding in from people that I had never even met. It meant everything to me because during that time I was really feeling so alone in the world.

But even in the midst of the outpouring of support, there was also a wave of hate that came.

I received multiple ugly messages from other mast cell activation syndrome and tick-borne disease patients who felt that my family starting a fundraiser to help get me to the appropriate doctor and get proper medical treatment was, in their words, "selfish" and stated that I "should be ashamed" because there were too many other patients out there who needed help besides me.

I'm not sure why they felt they had the right to message a sick and dying person things like this, but it didn't stop there! During that time, my now ex-stepfather-in-law was upset that my amazing mother-in-law was trying her best to help us in whatever way she could with the fundraiser. She told him, "She is dying. We are trying to save her life." And his reply to her was "Everyone has to die sometime." Other hateful comments were that I was making up my illness in order to start a GoFundMe to make money, which was very untrue. I mean, I was just in the hospital, paralyzed and dying. The GoFundMe itself raised just a hair over $6,000, which was beyond a blessing and an answered prayer because of all the medical costs that we were facing that my insurance would not pay for, such as seeing the mast cell and tick-borne disease specialist, having the proper testing ordered, trying different medical treatments and traveling out of state to try different treatment options. That's only a fraction of some of the costs we faced, and if we're being honest, it has taken over $100,000 out of pocket just to get me to the point where I am now.

This was just a glimpse of some of the hate that came my way. At first it really got to me, and all I could do was cry. I couldn't comprehend why in the world someone would ever treat someone as if their life didn't matter. The reason why I couldn't understand that concept is because I could never do that myself. All life is beyond precious to me, even the ones who acted as if mine wasn't worth saving. This eventually led us to closing the fundraiser down because I just couldn't tolerate the hate being thrown my way.

During that time my family had also reached out to over 250+ churches in Alabama, including a personal church, praying that they may offer a glimmer of hope, whether it came in the form of words of wisdom along with prayer through a phone call or simply a card in the mail or even a small donation toward the mountain of medical bills and treatment costs we faced.

Astonishingly, when it came down to it we only heard back from three of the churches that they reached out to, and I am forever grateful to those three churches, as you couldn't even begin to imagine the amount of pride I had to lay down to even ask for prayers and help in the first place. I had to truly humble myself like never before, and for them to take the time to show the love of Christ in a moment in my life where I was most vulnerable spiritually had a great impact on me because I think if I wouldn't have at least received those three replies of acknowledgement out of 250+ churches, I would have lost a little hope altogether.

Someone in my family did receive a call from their church, but it wasn't the call you would expect to receive from a ministry, as it was only the church secretary calling to ask my family member if what we said in the letter was true. My family member nicely informed whoever called from the church that we were asking for churches to come together in prayer about the situation and also raising funds for medical costs. The lady then said, "Okay, just wanted to make sure you knew about the fundraiser," and she hung up. My family member then waited to hear back from them, as this certain family member was very active in supporting the church, but the church never reached out again. This specific church knew I had been sick for some time, as I had been on the prayer list a while back as I began to slowly decline. My family member looked at me and said, "I am a little hurt. If it would have been the preacher's immediate family, the outcome would have been different." I was left speechless by the statement because I felt bad that this person had experienced that, but I couldn't help but wonder if the statement was true.

Now, I know that there is a lot going on in the world and many churches are busy, but it was just simply mind-blowing to us that we only heard back from that small a number of ministries, not to mention the response that my family was met with from their own church.

Growing up in the Christian faith, you're taught to always reach out to the church when you are sick or in need so that the elders of the church may pray for you and, if possible, offer a lending hand as Jesus would no matter who it may be. So, since I'd had that kind of upbringing, I had thought that more ministers of the church would have reached out to at least offer prayer to someone who was going through such hell on earth. I had never seen this side of the Christian church before. It made me wonder just how many people there are reaching out to the church, praying for even a small word from God or for a shred of hope, only to be ignored or turned away. It reminded me of the Bible story you often hear as a child of the Good Samaritan.

It starts off by Jesus being asked, "What was the greatest commandment of them all?"

Jesus replied, "To love God with all your heart, soul and mind." He then went on to say the second greatest would be to "Love your neighbor as yourself."

He was then immediately asked, "Who counts as a neighbor?"

Jesus then replied with a parable.

In this parable, Jesus described a man who had been robbed, stripped naked of his clothing and beaten almost to death, then left lying on the side of the road, as if his life meant nothing.

Jesus then went on to say that a priest was traveling down this same road where this horrible attack happened. The priest saw the man lying on the side of the road dying, but instead of helping, the priest turned a blind eye and kept walking by the man.

Soon after the priest had passed, Jesus said that a Levite followed down the same road and the Levite saw the man naked and beaten in the road, but much like the priest, the Levite acted as if he hadn't seen the man and kept walking, leaving him for dead just as the priest had done.

Finally, Jesus describes a glimmer of hope in this dying man's life. A Good Samaritan begins to travel down the road, where he then sees the dying man lying on the side of the road. Without any hesitation the Good Samaritan rushes over to the man in need, showing him compassion. He looks at his wounds and takes out his wine, oil and bandages to clean and cover his wounds. He then picks him up and takes him to an inn, where he tells the innkeeper to do what he has to do to take care of the man and not to worry about the cost because he would come back and cover any additional cost when he came back through town.

Jesus then asked the man, "Which one of these three men do you think proved to be a neighbor to the dying man?"

The man replied, "The one that showed the dying man mercy."

Jesus then said, "You go and do likewise."

Instead of looking at the situation negatively, I chose to learn how to shine Christ's light the right way from the experience. It is really simple: we have to be the Good Samaritan, showing kindness and mercy in our everyday lives. Kindness is everything, and strangers from all over the world with completely different backgrounds helped show me just how powerful the simple act of kindness can truly be.

Showing people they are not alone is monumental, and just a single acknowledgment can mean a world of difference to someone who already feels abandoned in the world. I discovered that I do not want to be a normal Christian if that just means sitting on a pew every week and not reaching out to the lost, dying world, especially when they are reaching out to me.

Honestly, I do not mean for that to sound harsh, so please do not take it that way because I believe the true church does amazing things, and I know even with all of their flaws Jesus still thinks they're golden just like He thinks you and I both are. But after seeing the things that I have seen, it leads me to wonder who most churches are—the Priest, the Levite or the Good Samaritan?

I mention this with love to bring awareness to the church that we may be missing the mark by turning people away. When the sick, dying and hurting are reaching out to us, whether it be through a letter, a phone call or even in person, we should never ignore them. What would it hurt to write a simple encouraging letter back?

Did you know a simple letter can change someone's life? And if it's someone who is on the verge of taking their life because they feel there is no other way out, then a simple sheet of paper with an encouraging message could save their life because they wouldn't feel so alone! They would know that somewhere out there someone took the time to care!

To be truthful, the rate of suicide is high in the tick-borne disease and/or mast cell activation syndrome community. As a matter of fact, it is the number-one killer in patients with Lyme disease. I have personally lost multiple friends who were suffering from these illnesses to suicide this past year alone and have even seen patients searching for medically assisted suicide! Most of them did not have a great support system at home. A few of them had reached out to their churches, but because their illnesses caused them to be homebound, they didn't feel like they had support from their churches either. Over time it felt as if they were forgotten about, like an "out of sight, out of mind" kind of thing. Lack of a good support system is all too common in these communities as well as in other chronically ill communities.

Through observing other patients as well as instances throughout my own battle, I've come to learn that the people you thought would be there for you sometimes turn a blind eye.

I've seen families, including my own, completely ignore their so-called loved one, ignoring their cries for help while they're slowly dying, thinking that these illnesses are made up in their head, even though there is a mountain of medical evidence to back up their claim. The sad part is, I have seen these same family members crying at their loved one's funerals, saying they wish they would have done more.

I have seen family members add ingredients that they know their loved one reacts to in their food without them knowing just to "test" if their loved one was truly reacting to it or if "it was in their head," causing their loved one to experience a reaction all so they could test and see it with their own eyes.

I have seen lifelong friends disappear without a trace, and I have even seen many spouses give up hope, leaving who was supposed to be the love of their life to fight for their life alone while they sought comfort in another's arms.

I've seen the medical community turn patients away, offering no help or labeling the patient as crazy, and I have seen churches turn a blind eye as well.

It's time for this ruthless cycle to end, and that begins with us!

There is an entire world of people out there who are fighting for their lives and who want to feel like their lives matter. They just want to know that there is a purpose for them, that the suffering will end and that through it all they are loved and not abandoned in the world.

If someone is truly wanting to make a difference in the world, then this itself should be one of the main parts of anyone's ministry—and life, for that matter. If you don't have funds to help financially, that doesn't matter, as you can help someone by being there! What matters is that you acknowledged someone in need and you didn't look the other way, because in just showing compassion you proved to be the Good Samaritan in the only way that you could, and that kind of kindness will never go unnoticed, especially in the eyes of God.

If you're reading this and are going through a similar situation with suicidal thoughts because of the pain, please know that there is always another way even when it seems like all hope is lost. I know firsthand just how desperate someone can be to feel relief by stopping the pain, whether physical or emotional, but I can promise you that taking your own life is not the answer no matter how great the pain may be. You're not alone; you're treasured, and every breath you breathe is a miracle.

Your smile can brighten any room, and you're truly needed in this world. You have a light like no other, and at the right timing you're going to shine as bright as the sun. Just hang on, because even after the worst of storms the sun will always rise to shine again. You have a purpose. I may not be able to tell you what it is, but I can tell you that the world is a better place with you in it.

I learned at the end of the day that maybe I am just not meant to be inside of a church building, and I think that I am okay with that. As long as I have Jesus by my side, I know I can conquer anything. Even if that means I fall down, I know He will always be there to pick me back up again.

While all of this torturous battle was happening, all I had was my faith and my family to keep me going. I had been dying a very slow, painful death from starvation because of my body rejecting foods, and I was literately hanging on by a thread with the thought of death sounding pretty appealing at the time.

All I knew to do was hold on to the helm of His garment as tight as I possibly could and reassure myself of His promises, but my faith kept being tested at the time because not only was I having to reassure myself, but I was also having to reassure other Christians that I had faith.

What do I mean by that? Well, it may be shocking to know, but when you're sick and someone prays for you over and over, not only do you have to reassure yourself that God still has you in His hands, but you also have to reassure all the others who are praying for you that He does, because when there is no change in a situation they will start to question God for themselves, asking why He has yet to intervene. It eventually will start to feel like a burden to people, which typically will cause them to fade away from your life all because they do not comprehend why bad things can happen to good people.

Then I have encountered people who had seen my story online and wanted to pray for me. I am all for prayer because I believe prayer works and I can use all the prayers I can get, but in these specific situations their prayers left me feeling very down and bad about myself. You see, these people would recognize me, walk up, grab me and began praying while telling me that God hasn't healed me yet because I didn't have enough faith.

Supposedly, I was to ignore all the symptoms I was going through, confess that I was healed and live life as a normal person would, and then God would heal me if I truly believed. While I fully believe in confessing positive things, this just wasn't the case here, and it wasn't because I didn't have enough faith, because Jesus Himself said, "If you had the faith the size of a mustard seed…" Have you seen a mustard seed? If not, Google it—they are pretty dang small!

I mean, imagine telling a lame person to get up out of his or her wheelchair and walk instantly in the name of Jesus and then nothing happens! It can affect both parties' faith, but I have personally come to learn that some miracles take time and may not happen in an instant like we would hope for, but we must learn that situations like this should be handled with care. We should never get in the habit of blaming someone for things that are out of their control.

I've also had the pleasure of people telling me that there was a demon inside of me causing all of my issues and that all I had to do was rebuke it in the name of Jesus.

Statements such as this can be very harmful because here I am, hanging onto Jesus with all of my might, filled with His Holy Spirit and goodness, fighting for my life and praying my heart out for God to save me with every ounce of energy that I could muster up, already rebuking every sickness and disease in His name, only to be told by other Christians that there was a demon living inside of me.

Sometimes bad things happen in life and attacks can come our way, but that doesn't mean that someone is possessed by a demon just because they are sick.

We must do better when it comes to our words and actions in the lives of others. Our words have the power to build someone up or tear someone down, and I truly believe if you really want to make a difference in the world and help show Jesus's mercy, kindness, and love in someone's life, the most important things to do are simple: Offer a smile and a gentle hand. When offering prayer for someone, be careful with your words, lifting the person up instead of saying prayers that may make them question their faith if they do not receive an instant healing. And most of all, never think you're better than someone else, because one thing is for sure: Jesus loves the beggar and prostitute on the street corner just as much as He loves you.

I can promise you any effort you put into letting that person know they are not alone will mean everything, even if it is just a tiny brief note in the mail. Always keep in mind that just because the person's healing doesn't happen instantly doesn't mean that you or the person you are praying for has done anything wrong. Sometimes life just isn't fair. Sometimes miracles take time.

Chapter 14

The Here and Now

Going back to where I am today, thanks to the help of amazing people, I was able to be seen by and am still under the care of a very knowledgeable and compassionate mast cell and tick-borne disease specialist.

Not only did this specialist order the proper testing needed, but she also found that I had a previous Lyme disease infection that was also cause by the tick bite!

She discovered this by ordering the Igenex Lyme test, because the standard Lyme test most doctors order often yields false negatives. The Igenex test also tests for other strains of Lyme bacteria that the standard testing does not even test for.

I'm sure you could imagine the shock that fell upon my face as she told me that the doctors before her missed yet again another tick-borne disease! All I could picture was the infectious disease doctor at what was supposed to be the state's best teaching hospital looking me in the eyes with an attitude and telling me the CDC should have never sent me to him because there is no such thing as Lyme disease or Rocky Mountain spotted fever in Alabama.

I'm not sure how a medical institute can legally get away with turning patients away because they think that there is no such thing as tick-borne diseases in the state of Alabama, and believe me, I am far from the first person to have this problem. It turns out that a large majority of people have had the same experience with the infectious disease department of this teaching medical hospital, and it leads me to wonder how many patients are getting worse because of it as I did because they are told that Lyme disease and Rocky Mountain spotted fever are not in their state? The scary part is, like I mentioned before, this is a teaching hospital!

Here's a kicker for you: the CDC estimates that there are 300,000+ Lyme disease infections in the U.S. each year, and that's not mentioning that it's spreading throughout the rest of the world. I don't know about you, but that sure sounds like a pandemic to me! Why is this not being discussed more in the medical community? Why are patients being told it's not in their area when there is clearly evidence showing otherwise?

I recently came across an article stating that the U.S. Pentagon had recently been told to investigate claims that Lyme disease in the U.S. was actually caused by an escaped experimental bioweapon from the Cold War between the years of "1950 and 1975."

Whether or not these claims are true, it is definitely intriguing and worth investigating. You can read more about these claims in the book *Bitten: The Secret History of Lyme Disease and Biological Weapons* written by Kris Newby and the book *Lab 257: The Disturbing Story of the Government's Secret Plum Island Germ Laboratory* written by Michael Christopher Carroll. Both books discussed programs that were designed by the government to research ways that arthropods could be used to spread bio-agents.

Research in these books suggest a military experiment gone wrong could have led to the sudden increase of Lyme disease in the U.S. Both books should make a very interesting read, and I'm curious to see how the Pentagon's investigation unfolds, but I'm not holding my breath, as I'm sure that's just not something anyone—much less a country—would be willing to admit to.

The good news was that my body appeared to have defeated the Lyme disease infection on its own, but the bad part is I developed mast cell activation syndrome in the midst of fighting the Lyme disease, Rocky Mountain spotted fever and the alpha-gal syndrome.

The specialist said that she wanted to run a mycotoxin test to check for mold exposure, and surprisingly the results revealed that I had been exposed to high levels of mold toxins, which can cause patients with mast cell activation syndrome and tick-borne disease to become worse!

She also discovered that my husband and son, after getting bitten by several ticks, both tested positive for old infections for tick-borne disease, and my son tested positive for West Nile! They both tested positive for Alpha-gal syndrome, so they have had to make some major life changes. One thing I will say is that Alpha-gal syndrome presented itself differently in all three of us. I may experience anaphylaxis; my husband may have high blood pressure, migraines, joint pains and hives; and our son may break out in a facial rash, develop canker sores in his mouth, a runny nose, GI reactions and develop small tics when exposed to any type of mammalian animal byproducts or meats.

It turned out that I became allergic to the place where we were living. The company who had remodeled the house had used a chemical scent paste under the flooring throughout the whole house, and I could no longer stay inside without experiencing symptoms.

Luckily, we had just bought a new travel trailer for me to have a safe way to travel out of state to the mast cell specialist in Colorado, so we decided to temporarily move into the travel trailer while we were in the process of trying to build a new home in a safe environment for me sometime in the future.

It has taken two very long years of physical therapy, but I can walk again, thank God! However, it was not an easy feat I was not able to go into a rehab for physical therapy because they could not accommodate my needs, leaving me to have to manage my therapy at home. I started off by holding myself up with the use of a handicap bar. When I first began, I could only tolerate holding myself up on my feet for about a minute or two before I could no longer handle the pain.

I can recall the first time I saw my lower body in the mirror during this time. I had just gotten the strength to pull myself up out of the wheelchair and look into the bathroom mirror. I can remember the horror on my face gazing back at me, as I did not realize just how much muscle atrophy I had endured.

My legs looked like a picture you would have seen in school of the holocaust victims. My knees appeared to be huge while the rest of my legs were just skin and bones with no muscle on them. I instantly went into uncontrollable tears. My husband heard me crying from the next room over and rushed in to see what was wrong. I remember the feeling of him just holding me, reminding me how beautiful that I was and that everything was going to be okay.

Over time, I was able to slowly increase my standing time from one minute to five minutes and then ten minutes. Once I was able to get to the point where I could stand for a short period of time, I then had to practice letting go of the bar to try to keep my balance. As I mastered that, I then had to learn how to pick my legs up all the way to take steps with the help of a walker.

Once I could walk on my own, I purchased the DB Method machine, and it helped me to regain balance as well as work muscles that I hadn't felt in years. I know that all of this may seem minor, but I can assure you that this was no simple task, and it has taken years to get my balance, strength and muscle mass back to the point where it is now.

I still suffer from nerve damage in my feet, which causes loss of feeling in certain spots, but I can walk and wiggle my toes! I actually went not too long ago for my first walk down a nature trail for the first time in over four years! I now have a full bucket list of things in life that I want to do. Of course, they all involve being out in nature, as I don't do too well in town, but I am looking forward to experiencing them!

I believe in miracles because I am living one every day. I learned that some miracles may come instantly and some may take time. Just never give up on your faith; hang on to those dreams, love, because it can become a reality. If you were to have told me three years ago that I would be alive right now, writing a book and making amazing new memories with my family, honestly I probably would have laughed at you because I was told by the doctors I most likely wouldn't make it to my 29th birthday, which at that point was only four months away!

I was lying in the hospital bed, planning my own funeral, making private videos for my son, husband and family to have as my last words to them—and not only to them but also to my future daughter-in-law and hopefully future grandkids. I had so much to say to everyone, and I had come to the reality I would not make it.

That's until God put a little hope back into my life. You know, I really can't say enough about that special nutritionist who helped save my life, and it wasn't only the nutritional knowledge I am referring to; it was the Jesus in him as well.

Him spending hours in my lonely hospital room listening to me cry, all the while showing the love of Christ, encouraged me to hope again and reassured me that Jesus was still there. We talked about confessing good things every day, which at that point I had been lacking, so I corrected myself and I eventually started to confess every day that I would walk again in the name of Jesus and that I would live and not die. The doctor not only helped my body physically, but he went above and beyond to help my spirit as well, and I will forever be grateful to him for that.

As far as my life right now, I am settled in my little bubble, just trying to help educate others as well as trying to show that I care in the little ways that I can and cherishing each day as if it's my last because living with this condition, you never know what tomorrow will bring, and sometimes you wonder if there will even be a tomorrow.

I am looking forward to our future home that is hopefully in the works, and I am excited about having enough space to try to grow different organic foods to try out. The place where I am at now gives me the chance to breathe fresh air without breathing in chemical triggers that burn my lungs—and, oh, how it feels so good just to be able to take in a deep breath of fresh air.

We also have a well now, which is simply AMAZING! Having the freedom to walk to the kitchen sink, filling your cup with cold fresh water and being able to drink it is a liberating feeling with a sense of gratefulness. Not only can I drink the well water where I'm at now, but I can also take a nice hot long shower without breaking out in red itchy patches, and I no longer have facial breakouts from the added chemicals in city water!

I have good and bad days; I just choose to focus on the good ones. On my good days I am able to take time to play with my son and watch him grow up, which is such a blessing because I thought I would miss out on it all. Hopefully I will meet my future daughter-in-law in person instead of her meeting me through an old recorded video.

I have since founded a mast cell activation syndrome and tick-borne disease resource organization in hopes that others may find the information and medical resources that they need to get speedy diagnoses. That way, they do not have to wait years like I did before being properly diagnosed and treated.

I also hope to bring awareness to the fact that medical cannabis is not a bad thing; in fact, without it I would not be here, and I think that my life as well as countless others' lives are worth saving, don't you?

I love God, I try my best to treat others with kindness and I do my best every day, but in some people's eyes—even Christians'—the fact that I need medical cannabis to help keep me alive causes them to instantly look down upon me instead of taking the time to get to know me for themselves.

I once sat through a sermon where the preacher was attacking marijuana. He said that he often hears people quoting Genesis 1:29 in favor of marijuana.

"God said, see, I have given you every herb that yields seed which is on the face of all the earth and every tree whose fruit yields seed; to you it shall be your food" (Genesis 1:29).

After quoting this scripture himself, he went on to preach that "God had created poison ivy too, so that must mean it's okay to smoke too!" He then asked the crowd sitting in the pews if they would smoke poison ivy! As if marijuana, an herb that has been scientifically proven to help medically could even compare to poison ivy! That sounds absolutely ridiculous, doesn't it? There really are Christians who are strongly against this God-given medicine!

It's a sad truth, and the saddest part is I never asked for this. I never knew that medical cannabis would be the medical treatment option helping my mast cells to stabilize the most—actually I would have never even dreamed of it—but guess what? Here I am, and another mind-blower is that I was crying out to God when I found this treatment option. Now, I know to some that's a touchy subject, but to me God used medical cannabis to save my life, and for that I am eternally grateful for Him designing our bodies with cannabinoid receptors on our mast cells. His intelligent design, His plant, His medicine saved my life.

~~The End~~

The Awakening.

Citations

Small-Howard, A. L., Shimoda, L. M., Adra, C. N., & Turner, H. (2005). Anti-inflammatory potential of CB1-mediated cAMP elevation in mast cells. The Biochemical journal, 388(Pt 2), 465–473. https://doi.org/10.1042/BJ20041682

Differential Roles of CB1 and CB2 Cannabinoid Receptors in Mast Cells
Maria-Teresa Samson, Andrea Small-Howard, Lori M. N. Shimoda, Murielle Koblan-Huberson, Alexander J. Stokes, Helen Turner
The Journal of Immunology May 15, 2003, 170 (10) 4953-4962; DOI: 10.4049/jimmunol.170.10.4953

CPSIA information can be obtained
at www.ICGtesting.com
Printed in the USA
LVHW040449180122
708503LV00003B/198